Wound and Skin Care

Editors

XIAOHUA ZHOU
CASSANDRA BUCHANAN RENFRO

PHYSICAL MEDICINE AND REHABILITATION CLINICS OF NORTH AMERICA

www.pmr.theclinics.com

Consulting Editor
SANTOS F. MARTINEZ

November 2022 • Volume 33 • Number 4

ELSEVIER

1600 John F. Kennedy Boulevard • Suite 1800 • Philadelphia, Pennsylvania, 19103-2899

http://www.theclinics.com

PHYSICAL MEDICINE AND REHABILITATION CLINICS OF NORTH AMERICA Volume 33, Number 4
November 2022 ISSN 1047-9651, 978-0-323-84892-3

Editor: Megan Ashdown
Developmental Editor: Diana Grace Ang

Reprints. For copies of 100 or more of articles in this publication, please contact the Commercial Reprints Department, Elsevier Inc., 360 Park Avenue South, New York, NY 10010-1710. Tel.: 212-633-3874; Fax: 212-633-3820; E-mail: reprints@elsevier.com.

Physical Medicine and Rehabilitation Clinics of North America (ISSN 1047-9651) is published quarterly by Elsevier Inc., 360 Park Avenue South, New York, NY 10010-1710. Months of issue are February, May, August, and November. Business and Editorial Offices: 1600 John F. Kennedy Blvd., Suite 1800, Philadelphia, PA 19103-2899. Customer Service Office: 3251 Riverport Lane, Maryland Heights, MO 63043. Periodicals postage paid at New York, NY and additional mailing offices. Subscription price per year is $332.00 (US individuals), $905.00 (US institutions), $100.00 (US students), $377.00 (Canadian individuals), $932.00 (Canadian institutions), $100.00 (Canadian students), $477.00 (foreign individuals), $932.00 (foreign institutions), and $210.00 (foreign students). Foreign air speed delivery is included in all *Clinics* subscription prices. All prices are subject to change without notice. **POSTMASTER:** Send address changes to *Physical Medicine and Rehabilitation Clinics of North America*, Customer Service Office: Elsevier Health Sciences Division, Subscription Customer Service, 3251 Riverport Lane, Maryland Heights, MO 63043. **Customer Service: 1-800-654-2452 (US). From outside of the United States, call 314-447-8871. Fax: 314-447-8029. E-mail: JournalsCustomer Service-usa@elsevier.com (for print support); JournalsOnlineSupport-usa@elsevier.com (for online support).**

Physical Medicine and Rehabilitation Clinics of North America is indexed in *Excerpta Medica, MEDLINE/ PubMed (Index Medicus), Cinahl, and Cumulative Index to Nursing and Allied Health Literature.*

Contributors

CONSULTING EDITOR

SANTOS F. MARTINEZ, MD, MS
Physical Medicine and Rehabilitation, Assistant Professor, Department of Orthopaedic Surgery and Biomedical Engineering, University of Tennessee College of Medicine, Campbell Clinic Orthopaedics, Memphis, Tennessee, USA

EDITORS

XIAOHUA ZHOU, MD
Department of Physical Medicine and Rehabilitation, UAB Heersink School of Medicine, The University of Alabama at Birmingham, Birmingham, Alabama, USA

CASSANDRA BUCHANAN RENFRO, DO
Department of Physical Medicine and Rehabilitation, UAB Heersink School of Medicine, The University of Alabama at Birmingham, Birmingham, Alabama, USA

AUTHORS

SARAH ASHOURI, MSN, CRNP
Nurse Practitioner, Trauma Burn Surgery, The University of Alabama at Birmingham, Birmingham, Alabama, USA

MALLORY BECKER, RN, BSN, CWCN, CRRN
Elevance Health Companies, Indianapolis, Indiana, USA; Robley Rex VA Medical Center, Fort Knox CBOC, Fort Knox, Kentucky, USA

NING CAO, MD
Attending Physician, Clinical Director of MossRehab Stroke Rehabilitation Program, MossRehab, Elkins Park, Pennsylvania, USA

CATHY H. CARVER, MS, PT, ATP/SMS
UAB Spain Rehabilitation Center, Birmingham, Alabama, USA

EMANUELE CEREDA, MD, PhD
UOC Dietetica e Nutrizione Clinica, Fondazione IRCCS Policlinico San Matteo, Viale Golgi, Pavia, Italy

WEI F. CHEN, MD, FACS
Professor, Department of Plastic Surgery, Center for Lymphedema Research and Reconstruction, Cleveland Clinic, Cleveland, Ohio, USA

ELIZABETH DAY DECHANT, BSN, RN, CWOCN, CFCN
Certified Wound Ostomy Continence Nurse, Children's of Alabama, Birmingham, Alabama, USA

KATHLEEN H. FITZGERALD, PT, DPT, NCS
Department of Physical Therapy, Faulkner University, Montgomery, Alabama, USA

JENNIFER HUTTON, MS, RN, CNS, CWCN, CRRN
Rocky Mountain Regional VA Medical Center, Aurora, Colorado, USA

MATTHEW J. JOHNSON, DPM, AACFAS
Assistant Professor, Department of Orthopaedic Surgery, UT Southwestern Medical Center, Dallas, Texas, USA

LYNDSAY A. KANDI, BS
Division of Plastic and Reconstructive Surgery, Department of Surgery, Mayo Clinic, Phoenix, Arizona, USA

MERRINE KLAKEEL, DO
Assistant Professor, Physical Medicine and Rehabilitation, UT Southwestern Medical Center, Dallas, Texas, USA

REBECCA KNACKSTEDT, MD, PhD
Department of Plastic Surgery, Center for Lymphedema Research and Reconstruction, Cleveland Clinic, Cleveland, Ohio, USA

KAREN KOWALSKE, MD
Professor, Physical Medicine and Rehabilitation, UT Southwestern Medical Center, Dallas, Texas, USA

ERWIN A. KRUGER, MD
Division of Plastic and Reconstructive Surgery, Department of Surgery, Mayo Clinic, Phoenix, Arizona, USA

MICHAEL KWASNIEWSKI, MD
Clinical Director, Inpatient Amputation Rehabilitation Program, MossRehab, Elkins Park, Pennsylvania, USA

CHERYL ANDERSON LANE, DNP, FNP, CRRN, CWCN
Retired Nurse Practitioner and Certified Wound Care Nurse, Physical Medicine and Rehabilitation Department, UAB Spain Rehabilitation Center, Birmingham, Alabama, USA

MARY LITCHFORD, PhD, RDN, LD
President Case Software, CASE Software & Books, Greensboro, North Carolina, USA

BIANCA MARTINEZ, MD
Resident Physician, Temple/MossRehab Department of Physical Medicine and Rehabilitation, Philadelphia, Pennsylvania, USA

GEORGE MARZLOFF, MD
Attending Physician, Spinal Cord Injury, Assistant Professor, University of Colorado School of Medicine, Rocky Mountain Regional VA Medical Center, Aurora, Colorado, USA

DANIELLE MITCHEL, MD
Resident, Physical Medicine and Rehabilitation, Temple University Hospital/MossRehab, Philadelphia, Pennsylvania, USA

DANIEL MOON, MD, MS
Attending Physician, Sheer Gait and Motion Analysis Laboratory and Motor Control Analysis Laboratory, MossRehab, Elkins Park, Pennsylvania, USA

NELLIE V. MOVTCHAN, MD
Division of Plastic and Reconstructive Surgery, Department of Surgery, Mayo Clinic, Phoenix, Arizona, USA

STACEY MULLIS, OTR/L, ATP
Clinical Marketing, Anthros, Waukesha, Wisconsin, USA

NANCY MUNOZ, DCN, MHA, RDN, FAND
Lecturer, University of Massachusetts, Amherst Chief, NFS VA Southern Nevada Healthcare System, Las Vegas, Nevada, USA

KAILA OTT, MS, ATP
Rocky Mountain Regional VA Medical Center, Aurora, Colorado, USA

INDIA C. RANGEL, BS
Mayo Clinic Alix School of Medicine, Scottsdale, Arizona, USA

KATHERINE M. RASPOVIC, DPM, FACFAS
Associate Professor, Department of Orthopaedic Surgery, UT Southwestern Medical Center, Dallas, Texas, USA

STEPHANIE RYDER, MD
Attending Physician, Spinal Cord Injury, Assistant Professor, University of Colorado School of Medicine, Rocky Mountain Regional VA Medical Center, Aurora, Colorado, USA

SCOTT SCHUBERT, MD
Spinal Cord Injury Provider, Section Chief, Assistant Professor, University of Colorado School of Medicine, Rocky Mountain Regional VA Medical Center, Aurora, Colorado, USA

NICOLE R. VAN SPRONSEN, MD
Division of Plastic and Reconstructive Surgery, Department of Surgery, Mayo Clinic, Phoenix, Arizona, USA

KARION GRAY WAITES, DNP, CRRN
Nurse Practitioner, Physical Medicine and Rehabilitation Department, UAB Spain Rehabilitation Center, Birmingham, Alabama, USA

DANE K. WUKICH, MD
Professor and Chair, Department of Orthopaedic Surgery, UT Southwestern Medical Center, Dallas, Texas, USA

Contents

> The skin's ability to function optimally is compromised when skin integrity is altered. The goals for skin management during rehabilitation include maintaining skin integrity, avoiding skin injury, providing early intervention, and comprehensive education for long-term skin management. Assessment of the whole patient as well as the skin is essential. Common issues seen in rehabilitation such as aging skin, incontinence dermatitis, intertrigo/yeast, surgical wounds, and pressure injuries are addressed.

> Wound care in pediatrics is a specialized area of practice that requires consideration of factors unique to pediatric patients. With a slowly growing body of evidence to support treatment choices in this vulnerable population, it is critical that wound experts develop and oversee evidence-based skin care regimens and wound treatment practices. This article discusses some common issues in pediatric skin and wound care. A successful prevention or treatment plan is collaborative and addresses the developmental, physiologic, and social needs of the pediatric patient and their family. Conflicting plans of care and limited resources are frequent challenges.

> Pressure injuries (PIs) are a spectrum of localized tissue destruction that develops most often at a bony prominence. PIs are the result of a combination of extrinsic (eg, pressure, shear, friction, and moisture) and intrinsic (nutritional status, spasticity, decreased sensation, and vascular disease) factors. Given their complex etiology, management of PIs requires a multidisciplinary approach from a team of health care professionals. After addressing both extrinsic and intrinsic factors, local wound care is generally recommended for stages 1 to 2 PIs and surgical intervention for stages 3 to 4.

Many know that the wound care team consists of physicians and nurses with specialized training. Many may not know of physical therapists (PT) or occupational therapists (OT) with training in seating and wheeled mobility who address skin injuries in people who are full-time wheelchair users. PTs/OTs address the fit and use of their wheelchair to their body and look at their daily function while looking for causes of skin injury otherwise not seen and can help prevent them in the future. Therefore, this makes PTs and OTs with this expertise a valuable part of the wound care team.

A comprehensive, interdisciplinary wound care team is of great importance to the management of acute, chronic, and recurrent wounds. This management functions best for the patient when all members of the team are in regular discussion regarding the wound care plan, providing more efficient and timelier patient-centered care. This article reviews the roles of different disciplines in the management of wounds. These disciplines include rehabilitation physicians, wound care nurses, registered nurses and certified nursing assistants, surgical teams, specialists of infectious diseases and mental health, dieticians, and patients and caregivers. A case study is also provided.

Nutrition is an important component of health and well-being. A compromised nutritional status has been linked to increased risk for wound development, difficulty managing, and decreased wound healing rate. Malnutrition contributes to an immunocompromised system, reduced collagen synthesis, and diminished tensile strength during the wound healing process. This is why assessment and optimization of nutritional status should be incorporated as part of a comprehensive treatment plan for individuals with wounds. The nutrition care plan must include individualized interventions designed to address the individual's nutrition diagnosis. This article reviews the role of nutrition in wound prevention, management, and treatment.

Hyperbaric oxygen (HBO) is a Medicare-approved treatment for a variety of diagnoses including chronic nonhealing wounds and radiation necrosis. Hyperbaric oxygen therapy (HBOT) uses high pressures to saturate hemoglobin and dissolve oxygen into blood plasma to create a hyperoxemic environment to nourish and reverse local tissue injury caused by ischemia and hypoxemia. HBOT is expensive and not without risk; therefore, the underlying etiology for the presenting diagnosis must be adequately treated before starting HBO as an adjunct therapy to get maximum benefit.

A Stepwise Approach to Nonoperative and Operative Management of the Diabetic Foot Ulceration

Katherine M. Raspovic, Matthew J. Johnson, and Dane K. Wukich

There are multiple factors that lead to the development of the diabetic foot ulceration (DFU). The ultimate goal when treating DFU is to prevent amputation. Initial therapy should include debridement, maintaining a healthy wound environment, and offloading. In the setting of infection or a non-healing DFU, surgical intervention may be necessary. The goals of this article are to discuss the key aspects of the initial examination, standard nonoperative treatment, and the operative treatment options for patients with DFU.

Shoe and Bracing Considerations for the Insensate Foot: Shoe considerations for diabetic foot

Daniel Moon, Ning Cao, and Bianca Martinez

Diabetic individuals with peripheral neuropathy are at risk for the development of foot ulcers due to musculoskeletal abnormalities and abnormal loading in the gait cycle leading to elevated plantar pressures. To prevent diabetic foot ulcers, practitioners should regularly screen patients for the presence of neuropathy as well as neuroarthropathies and prescribe the appropriate shoes and orthotics based on the best available clinical evidence. Although not widely available, there is potential for data-driven customization of orthotics and shoe wear based on plantar pressure data to prevent the development of diabetic foot ulcers more effectively, and ultimately prevent lower limb amputations.

Post Amputation Skin and Wound Care

Michael Kwasniewski and Danielle Mitchel

Management of the post amputation wound and skin is an individualized and evolving process. Although no consensus recommendations are available, optimal wound healing occurs with a dressing that provides the appropriate level of moisture, and management of edema, and can assist in contracture prevention and limb protection. Management of comorbid conditions and complications that might impede healing, as well as nutritional optimization help promotes wound closure. A faster time to heal increases the opportunity and likelihood of prosthetic fitting and use, working toward improved functional independence.

An Introduction to Burns

Sarah Ashouri

Burn injuries are often devastating and result in lifelong sequelae such as scar contracture, pain, and disfiguration with care beginning at the time of injury and extending through discharge to outpatient care where the largely becomes scar and mobility optimization. The Physical Medicine and Rehab (PM&R) team are integral in improving the quality of life of burn patients during and following recovery. This article functions to provide a brief overview of burn care to the non-burn specialized audience, discuss select advanced burn interventions, and provide an introduction to the role of PM&R in the life of a burn patient.

 Video content accompanies this article at http://www.pmr.theclinics. com.

The decision on whom to offer surgical interventions for lymphedema requires collaboration and input from all involved specialists and should address patients' expectations, invasiveness of procedures, and disease severity. There is no consensus on what constitutes success or failure of complex decongestive therapy and when to pursue surgical intervention. Surgery has the potential to fundamentally affect the pathophysiology of the disease state and can be a powerful tool when used correctly. The dogma of which surgery to offer for a given clinical situation has been undergoing revision and is an area of ongoing research.

Technological advances are incorporated into wound care management to enhance prevention through specialty mattresses and pressure mapping, assessment using modern imaging, and treatment with dressings and active therapies. We review specific equipment and evidence-based practice in the context of managing pressure injuries in patients with spinal cord injury.

PHYSICAL MEDICINE AND REHABILITATION CLINICS OF NORTH AMERICA

SERIES OF RELATED INTEREST

Orthopedic Clinics
https://www.orthopedic.theclinics.com/
Neurologic Clinics
https://www.neurologic.theclinics.com/
Clinics in Sports Medicine
https://www.sportsmed.theclinics.com/

VISIT THE CLINICS ONLINE!
Access your subscription at:
www.theclinics.com

Foreword

A Recap on Basics

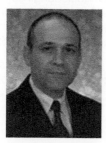

Santos F. Martinez, MD, MS
Consulting Editor

Skin functions as our largest organ system and provides many functions serving as a protective self-replenishing barrier/envelope with specialized sensory, excretory, and thermoregulatory qualities. Although there are related immunologic and metabolic functions, our mission in this issue focuses on pathologic condition that we encounter in the Rehabilitation patient, the potential pitfalls, and strategies and addresses these as a team. Our field inherently works with individuals who are limited from a wide array of conditions that disrupt one's existential homeostasis, affecting mobility and metabolic/nutritional and neurovascular systems in a wide range of ages and medical conditions. Success does not end with discharge from hospitalization but is a new beginning for a patient's survival with new challenges dependent on their mastering key elements and their transmission to family and other supportive personnel. The importance of skin and wound care has achieved its subspecialty appeal among diverse dedicated affiliated fields who find themselves with a common goal. As always, prevention goes a long way in preventing future complications, and therefore, initial risk inventories are paramount to identify individualized needs. An amputee unable to use his/her prosthesis or a spinal cord patient unable to use their wheelchair due to skin breakdown not only has a major impact on their ability to interact with society or work but also can result in a progressive multisystem decompensation. It becomes everyone's job from the initial assessment by the nursing assistant of the cachectic malnourished individual with high-risk bony prominences and the morbidly obese bed-bound incontinent patient to support a gifted surgeon who may have to revise a limb or provide skin grafts or a myotendinous flap. This obviously requires an "all-hands-on-deck" attitude with input from everyone. Well-established monitoring methods include serial photo and/or pressure mapping modalities, skin perfusion assessments, nutritional optimization, debridement with other modalities such as negative pressure wound approaches, and more recent use of biologics. Skin and wound

Phys Med Rehabil Clin N Am 33 (2022) xiii–xiv
https://doi.org/10.1016/j.pmr.2022.08.002
1047-9651/22/© 2022 Published by Elsevier Inc.

care serves one well in our field and will always have a major impact for our patients. We should never forget the basics.

Santos F. Martinez, MD, MS
Physical Medicine and Rehabilitation
Department of Orthopaedic Surgery and Biomedical Engineering
University of Tennessee College of Medicine
Campbell Clinic Orthopaedics
Memphis, TN 38104, USA

E-mail address:
smartinez@campbellclinic.com

Preface

We Take on the Business

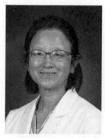 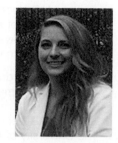

Xiaohua Zhou, MD   Cassandra Buchanan Renfro, DO
Editors

In Physical Medicine and Rehabilitation (PM&R) clinical practice, we too often encounter wound and skin care medical conditions with related complications. Whether the condition is the result of trauma, burn, surgery, pressure, diabetes, lymphedema, or from other medical consequences, we provide care beyond any required surgical intervention. PM&R offers unique interdisciplinary collaboration with doctors, physical and occupational therapists, nurses as well as orthotic and prosthetic professionals within the field. Together, PM&R professionals treat the person as a whole, which might include evaluations of nutrition, functional abilities, socioeconomic limitations, and psychological well-being. We have the training, experience, and passion to not only treat wounds and skin care but also prevent them in high-risk patient populations.

In this issue of *Physical Medicine and Rehabilitation Clinics of North America*, a group of outstanding and dedicated authors, who worked tirelessly during the difficult COVID-19 pandemic period, compiled the abundant evidence-based information on wound and skin care to serve as a valuable reference for physiatrists as well as other health care professionals. Within this issue, we aim to enhance the knowledge and our clinical capacity to effectively care for our patient populations, reduce unnecessary referrals, and ultimately offer our patients a better quality of life.

Phys Med Rehabil Clin N Am 33 (2022) xv–xvi
https://doi.org/10.1016/j.pmr.2022.08.001
1047-9651/22/© 2022 Published by Elsevier Inc.

pmr.theclinics.com

It is with great honor that we thank all contributors and practitioners for their ongoing contributions toward our goal.

Xiaohua Zhou, MD
The Department of Physical Medicine
and Rehabilitation
UAB Heersink School of Medicine
The University of Alabama at Birmingham
1717 6th Avenue South, Room R156
Birmingham, AL 35249, USA

Cassandra Buchanan Renfro, DO
The Department of Physical Medicine
and Rehabilitation
UAB Heersink School of Medicine
The University of Alabama at Birmingham
1717 6th Avenue South, Room R156
Birmingham, AL 35249, USA

E-mail addresses:
xzhou@uabmc.edu (X. Zhou)
cmrenfro@uabmc.edu (C.B. Renfro)

General Skin Issues in the Adult Rehabilitation Population

Cheryl Anderson Lane, DNP, FNP, CRRN, CWCN*,
Karion Gray Waites, DNP, CRRN

KEYWORDS

- Skin care • Assessment • Rehabilitation • Aging skin
- Incontinence-associated dermatitis • Intertrigo • Surgical wounds • Pressure injuries

KEY POINTS

- Thorough and consistent assessment of the skin is needed to identify the cause and location of altered skin and to begin preventive measures, early education, and intervention.
- Know which type of skin injury is being treated.
- Eliminate causative factors.
- Evaluate and treat the whole patient including the skin.

INTRODUCTION

Skin, the largest organ in the human body, has several functions including protection, immunity, thermoregulation, sensation, metabolism, and communication **Figs. 1–5**. The skin protects the body from experiencing excessive fluid loss, ultraviolet rays, both bacterial and viral pathogens, and mechanical assaults. In addition, the skin provides protection against aqueous and chemical assaults, as well as aids in providing immune protection against invading microorganisms. The skin acts as an environmental barrier and uses circulation and perspiration to provide thermoregulation for body temperature maintenance. Nerve fibers in the dermis and epidermis of the skin are sensitive to pain, touch, temperature, and pressure. The nerve receptors transmit the impulses to the brain where they are interpreted. Other responsibilities of the skin include the synthesis of vitamin D in the presence of sunlight, and as a covering on the face it is associated with communication and body image. Feelings of friendship, love, concern, and comfort can also be communicated with the

Physical Medicine and Rehabilitation Department, Spain Rehabilitation Center at UAB Hospitals, 1717 6th Avenue. South, Birmingham AL 35233, USA
* Corresponding author. 3227 Dundale Road, Hoover, AL 35216.
E-mail address: CHL42@aol.com

Phys Med Rehabil Clin N Am 33 (2022) 745–758
https://doi.org/10.1016/j.pmr.2022.06.001
1047-9651/22/© 2022 Elsevier Inc. All rights reserved.

pmr.theclinics.com

sensation of touch. An alteration in skin integrity compromises the skin's ability to provide these functions.[1,2]

Common diagnoses of patients in rehabilitation settings include stroke, spinal cord injury, orthopedic injury, and brain injury. These patients include the elderly, postsurgical, mobility impaired, cognitively impaired, and those with specialty devices. These patients often present with multiple risk factors for alteration in skin integrity and skin breakdown, which can negatively impact the ability to participate in therapies. The groups at highest risk are those who have been hospitalized for greater than 1 week, clients older than 65 years, those with a previous history of being residents in long-term care facilities, and those with spinal cord injury. Therefore, education about prevention of skin breakdown should be a part of an interdisciplinary plan of care. Strategies should be initiated and continued after rehabilitation to avoid additional compromise to skin integrity and to maintain the structure and function of the skin.[3] An overview including some of the more prevalent issues and/or concerns with this population including aging skin, incontinence dermatitis, intertrigo/yeast, surgical wounds, pressure injuries, wound healing, and dressings follows.

A consistent plan for skin assessment should be developed and maintained using validated tools and teams most effective for one's facility. Options include but are not limited to:

- Wound care associates
- Certified wound care nurses
- Rehabilitation nurse skin teams
- Interdisciplinary skin teams

DISCUSSION
Aging Skin

As a result of the following issues noted with aging skin, special precautions need to be taken during rehabilitation to avoid skin injury. The term *dermatoporosis* has been

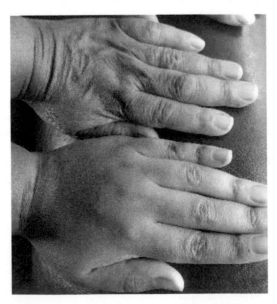

Fig. 1. Aging skin.

used since 2007 to describe the chronic, fragile skin noted with aging. Other identifying features of dermatoporosis include atrophic skin with solar purpura, white pseudoscars, skin tears or lacerations, and delayed healing. Dermatoporosis leaves the individuals susceptible to bleeding complications and cutaneous infections.[4]

As a person ages, the skin's ability to function optimally diminishes. This degenerative process is a result of internal and external factors. The number of growth factors and stem cells decline, the skin becomes increasingly fragile, and a wide range of issues occur including defective repair, deficient immunity, and vulnerability to infections. Although the entire pathologic basis for the aging process is poorly understood, it is confirmed that stem cell dysfunction, chronic disease, malnutrition, and sun exposure are contributing factors.[5]

Major risk factors for dermatoporosis start with advancing age, genetic susceptibility, corticosteroid use, and chronic actinic damage. Chronic renal failure, chronic obstructive pulmonary disease, impaired mental status, nutritional compromise, and history of skin tears are other risk factors identified with dermatoporosis.[4]

Some of the understood pathogenesis of aging skin notes the following:

- The epidermis becomes thinner with less definition of rete ridges as production of keratinocytes decline.[4]
- The dermis also declines in volume. The dermis is mainly composed of extracellular matrix (ECM), with fibroblasts, collagen, and elastin.[4]
- Hyaluronic acid within the ECM is needed to reduce friction but is also diminished resulting in increased vulnerability to skin tears.[4]
- Low levels of CD44, a cell surface receptor that stimulates keratinocyte production, is also noted resulting in skin atrophy.[4]
- Irregularity with matrix metalloproteinases (MMPs) also contributes to the breakdown of collagen and elastin in the dermis.[4]
- Ultraviolet radiation from sun exposure is well known to have negative impact on the skin with the worst being cutaneous malignancy. In fact, basal cell carcinoma is the most common skin cancer and is seen most often in the exposed skin of elderly individuals.[5]

Incontinence Dermatitis

Incontinence-associated dermatitis (IAD) is defined as inflammation and/or erosion of the skin in response to prolonged contact with urine or stool.[6] In the inpatient rehabilitation setting, individuals who are obese, who have had strokes, or have had spinal cord injuries are especially susceptible due to the incontinence that can occur with these diagnoses. In addition, individuals may develop short-term incontinence when physically dependent in the health care setting. Some contributing factors include medications, delays with the caregivers, problems with timely accessibility to commodes, inadequate staffing, and reluctance on the part of the patient to request assistance.[1] The key is to keep the skin clean and dry. Therefore, assessment of the skin as well as knowledge and implementation of bowel and bladder programs and breaking down barriers must occur to prevent incontinence from remaining on the skin.

The skin irritation from IAD occurs mostly due to chemical irritation from the pH changes that occur when urine and feces come in direct contact with the skin. The alkaline urine changes the skin's pH from acidic (pH < 7) to alkaline (pH > 7). Enzymes act on urea in urine making ammonia, which further increases the pH. Also, the alkaline urine promotes enzymatic activity of proteinases and lipases with fecal incontinence, causing even further skin erosion. Liquid stool typically has more digestive enzymes

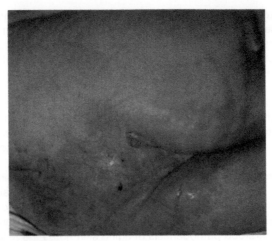

Fig. 2. Incontinence dermatitis.

than formed stool and causes more damage than formed stool.[7] Furthermore, prolonged moisture on the skin results in the epidermal layer of the skin being damaged, which makes it more susceptible to friction, shear, and pathogens such as *Candida albicans* and *Staphylococcus*.[7] IAD can be fairly widespread including the perineum, the labial folds, groin area, buttocks, scrotum, and gluteal fold and can extend to the inner and posterior thighs.[8]

Although additional research is needed for evidence-based management of IAD, a multinational group reviewed and evaluated available research and synthesized the information into best practice recommendations in 2009.[9] Best practice recommendations include

- Gentle skin cleansing
- Applying skin protectant
- Moisturizing
- Management of cutaneous candidiasis when needed
- Aggressive containment of urinary and fecal incontinence
- Recommendation of mild anti-inflammatory product in selected cases[9]

Cleaning the skin should occur as soon as possible. It is advised that the skin cleanser pH should range between 5.4 and 5.9, which is close to the pH of healthy skin. The pH of regular soap is typically 9.5 to 11 and can increase stratum corneum swelling, alter lipid rigidity, and may therefore be more damaging.[9] In addition, applying water alone can impair skin barrier function by causing an increase in transepidermal water loss. Also, infection control issues have been associated with the use of wash basins.[10] However, if soap and water are needed to remove dirt or irritants, gentle cleansing with a soft cloth to minimize friction damage is advised. Skin cleansers, including no-rinse skin cleansers, which are closer to the skin's pH, may reduce some of the adverse effects noted with soap and are preferable to soap and water. Some of these skin cleansers also have ingredients such as emollients and/or humectants that help restore or preserve optimal skin barrier functions.[9] Surfactants in skin cleansers help to reduce surface tension and allow soilage to be removed with minimal force. In addition, the skin cleanser wipes have a smoother surface and therefore less friction than using a rough washcloth. The expert panel advised that wherever possible, the use of no-rinse skin cleansers capable of removing incontinence should be used at least once daily and after each incontinent episode.[10]

A skin protectant needs to be used in the management of IAD as a preventative measure and also as a form of treatment. Another term for skin protectants is moisture barriers. Skin protectants form a barrier between the skin and any irritant such as urine or stool. As a form of treatment, the skin protectant is used to help resolve the IAD and allows the skin barrier to recover. There are many formulations including creams, ointments, pastes, lotions, and films. These products have varying main protective ingredients including petrolatum, zinc oxide, dimethicone, and acrylate terpolymer. However, the total formulation of the product determines its effectiveness, and they should be used as the manufacturers advice. Pros and cons of each product should be considered in selecting the best option for the patient.[10]

The next step after cleansing and protecting is restoring. Moisturizers help to restore the skin by reducing dryness and helping to restore the lipid matrix of the skin. A large selection of products is available with multiple components to restore the skin. It is also noted that some products have multiple uses such as cleaning, protecting, and restoring depending on the contents. Some contain a combination of emollients and humectants. Humectants draw in water and hold it in the stratum corneum and therefore are not advised on skin that is overhydrated. This is just one example of knowing the components of the products and using them as advised. So, a skin care regimen may not only use 3 separate items to cleanse, protect, and restore but also may use only 1 item such as continence care wipes that are designed to provide all 3 steps depending on availability, resources, and the needs of the patient.[10]

The most common skin infection with IAD is candidiasis, which can typically be treated topically. Antifungal creams and powders should be used with skin protectants. If the patient is not responding to treatment of C albicans, a sample should be obtained, and medical opinion sought for treatment of other Candida species and differentiation of other possible dermatologic conditions. Antimicrobials should only be used as needed and not as a prophylactic management strategy especially given the increase in antimicrobial resistance.[10] Evaluation of the treatment of IAD should be done regularly, and if no improvement in 3 to 5 days, the skin regimen should be reevaluated and adjusted and/or a referral to a specialist may be indicated. All patients with incontinence are at risk of IAD, and IAD is a contributing factor to the development of pressure injuries. Therefore, a skin care program with emphasis on prevention and early treatment is a wise use of resources to improve health care outcomes.[10]

Intertrigo/Yeast

Intertrigo dermatitis (ITD) occurs when moisture trapped in skin folds is subject to friction and results in inflammation. Immobility, obesity, deep skin folds, pendulous breasts, and diabetes are all risk factors for ITD. ITD can develop in any skin fold, but it has most notably been found in the axillary areas, inguinal folds, inframammary areas, under the abdominal or pubic panniculi, and under redundant skin after significant weight loss. Pruritis, pain, odor, and a mirror image rash are all noted with ITD. Owing to the trapped moisture, yeast is one of the more commonly associated skin infections associated with ITD.[1,8]

The stratum corneum layer of the skin becomes overhydrated by moisture that has not been absorbed or evaporated and is unable to glide on the opposing skin surfaces resulting in damage to the skin from friction. Also, there are many normal flora on the skin that can become pathogenic when skin is inflamed and denuded from maceration. Some of the normal flora include Staphylococcus epidermidis, Staphylococcus

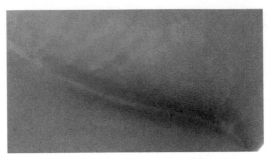

Fig. 3. Intertrigo/yeast.

aureus, Streptococcus pyogenes, corynebacteria, and mycobacteria.[8] Although the most common fungal infection is with *Candida,* ITD cultures have grown other pathogens such as *S aureus,* group A beta-hemolytic streptococcus, *Pseudomonas, Proteus mirabilis, Proteus vulgaris,* enterococci, and vancomycin-resistant enterococci[8]; this highlights the need to control ITD to avoid serious infections such as cellulitis or panniculitis.

Assessment, including a thorough visual inspection of all the skin surfaces, beneath folds, under axillae, neck creases, behind the knees, the inguinal fold, and interdigital areas, is vital for prevention and early intervention. Skin, including skin folds, should be kept clean and dry using a cleanser close to the skin's pH, cleaning gently and avoiding scrubbing. Skin folds should be patted dry, not rubbed, and fanned to dry, or a hairdryer should be used on cool setting. Additionally, loose-fitting, absorptive, clothing that wicks away moisture is advised. Various soaks, moisture wicking textiles, dressings, and absorptive powders have been advised, but products containing chlorhexidine gluconate, alcohol, or perfumes should be avoided due to the potential of further damage to the skin.[8]

Furthermore, skin that has become invaded with candidiasis should be treated with an antifungal agent. The antifungal agent will vary depending on the invading organism. As *Candida* growth is enhanced with the use of steroids, this should be used sparingly only as indicated. The ITD culture will determine more specific treatment of other invading organisms. Although rare, surgery to remove excess tissue has been done in some cases to promote dryness, reduce friction, and definitively manage intertriginal dermatitis.[8]

- Thoroughly assess the skin including all skin folds and creases
- Use cleanser close to skin pH
- Pat dry, do not rub
- Use appropriate treatment products that do not contain skin irritants
- Use antifungal agent if needed
- Wear loose-fitting, absorptive clothing

Surgical Wounds

Optimizing surgical wound care promotes healing without infection, dehiscence, or other complicating factors. Incisional or surgical wounds like all wounds progress through stages to heal completely.[1] The 3 major phases or stages of wound healing are the inflammatory phase, the proliferative phase, and the remodeling phase. Within these phases, hemostasis, inflammation, repair, and remodeling are the physiologic events that take place.[2] Surgical procedures are increasingly less invasive with

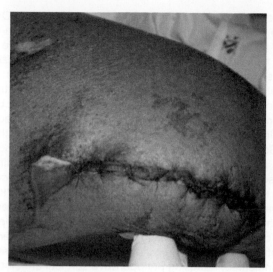

Fig. 4. Surgical wound.

arthroscopic and laproscopic procedures, but some surgeries are still done by an open incision. The open incision undergoes primary closure with sutures, staples, adhesive tapes, and skin adhesives. Surgical wounds can also be left open for delayed primary closure or healing by secondary intention. One reason why a surgical wound may be left open and closed later is a high bacterial load of greater than 10^5/g of tissue. After the bacterial load is reduced and a healthy wound bed is established, the wound can then be considered for closure.[1]

There are many methods of scoring wound healing and evaluating the healing process of a surgical wound. One generally accepted tool for evaluation of surgical wounds is ASEPSIS:

- A = Additional treatments such as antibiotics, drainage, or debridement
- S = Serous drainage
- E = Erythema
- P = Purulent exudate
- S = Separation of deep tissue
- I = Isolation of bacteria
- S = Prolonged inpatient stays over fourteen days.

Using this tool, the surgical wound is evaluated and given a score based on the proportion of wound affected and other characteristics. Based on the score, the wound is categorized in a range from satisfactory healing to severe wound infection. No matter what tool is used, the important thing is that the wound is assessed and that impediments to wound healing are addressed as early as possible. Some, but not all, impediments to surgical wound healing include hematomas or seromas, surgical wound infections, systemic infections, poor perfusion, nicotine use, nonviable tissue, malnutrition, obesity, diabetes, prior surgical site radiation, and steroid or immunosuppressive medications.[1]

Hospital-acquired surgical site infections (SSIs) have become such a health crisis that in 2008 the Centers for Medicare and Medicaid Services identified it as one of the first 8 conditions that were identified as preventable and would no longer receive reimbursement. The 3 types of SSIs are superficial incisional, deep incisional, and organ/space. In response to this health crisis, the World Health Organization, The American College of Surgeons and Surgical Infection Society, the Centers for Disease Control and Prevention, and other global organizations have publications on reducing SSIs. In these publications, the major focus is on optimizing the patient's condition before surgery and then continuing with best practices during and after surgery.[2] Some of the strongest recommendations included treatment of patients with known nasal carriage of S aureus. Hair should not be removed, but, if necessary, it should be cut only with a clipper. Shaving is strongly discouraged. When surgical antibiotic prophylaxis is advised, it should be administered within 120 minutes before incision. Scrubbing or a suitable alcohol-based hand rub should be used for surgical hand preparation before donning sterile gloves. Additionally, alcohol-based antiseptic solutions based on chlorhexidine gluconate surgical site skin preparation should be used. Surgical antibiotic prophylaxis administration should not be prolonged after the operation. Also, intubated patients should receive 80% fraction of inspired oxygen intraoperatively and for a period of 2 to 6 hours postoperatively if feasible.[11] Some of the issues addressed for postoperative concerns during which time the patient might be in the rehabilitation setting included promptly removing any drains when indicated, not using perioperative surgical antibiotics when a drain is present to prevent SSI, and avoiding the use of advanced dressing of any type over a standard dressing on a primarily closed wound for the purpose of preventing SSI.[11] Also, the use of topical antibiotics on closed surgical incisions is not supported scientifically.[1]

Regardless of what material is used to close a surgical wound, the wound should be assessed thoroughly including the dressing, epithelial resurfacing, wound closure, and any local changes indicative of surgical wound infection.[1] This assessment is especially important during the first 3 to 4 weeks postoperatively to detect problems early and intervene to avoid more severe postoperative complications. Some basic treatment of topical incisional care includes:

- Keep incisional area clean and dry without excessive exposure to moisture[1]
- Keep original dressing for the first 48 to 72 hours and clean with sterile water and aseptic technique if needed during that time[1]
- Shower after 48 to 72 hours if no drainage and incision intact[1]
- Remove sutures and staples based on their location (face: 3 to 5 days, scalp, chest, fingers hands, lower extremities: 7 to 10 days; back: 10 to 14 days)[1]
- Protect from sun exposure to prevent hyperpigmentation[1]
- Defer major complications with surgical incisional areas to the surgeon unless otherwise directed.

Pressure Injury/Device-Related Injury

Individuals with decreased mobility are especially vulnerable to pressure injuries, which can have significant negative outcomes including death.[12] The term *pressure injury* and the use of pressure injury staging should only be used in wounds that are due to pressure, and/or shear. There are separate staging guidelines for other types of wounds such as skin tears, burns, diabetic foot ulcers, venous leg ulcers, adhesive or tape injuries, and so on.

The definition and staging of pressure injuries was revised by the National Pressure Ulcer Advisory Panel in 2016 due to increased knowledge regarding the cause and for clarification of anatomic features associated with each stage.[13] Instead of ulcers, the new terminology uses the term injuries and denotes stages with Arabic numerals rather than Roman numerals. Pressure injury is defined as localized damage to the

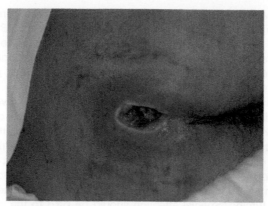

Fig. 5. Pressure injury.

skin and underlying soft tissue usually over a bony prominence or related to a medical or other device. The injury can present as intact skin or an open ulcer and may be painful. The injury occurs because of intense and/or prolonged pressure or pressure in combination with shear. The tolerance of soft tissue for pressure and shear may also be affected by microclimate, nutrition, perfusion, comorbid conditions, and condition of the soft tissue.[13]

The stages/categories for pressure injuries include stage 1, stage 2, stage 3, stage 4, unstageable full-thickness injury, deep tissue injury, device-related pressure injury, and mucosal membrane pressure injury. Briefly

- Stage 1 is intact skin with an area of nonblanchable erythema;
- Stage 2 is partial-thickness skin loss with exposed dermis;
- Stage 3 is full-thickness skin loss, where adipose tissue may be visible in the wound bed and granulation tissue and epibole (rolled edges) are often visible;
- Stage 4 is full-thickness skin and tissue loss with exposed or directly palpable fascia, muscle, tendon, ligament, cartilage, or bone in the ulcer;
- Unstageable full-thickness pressure injury has the wound bed obscured by slough or eschar and therefore the extent of tissue damage cannot be confirmed; when the wound bed is cleaned, it will be a stage 3 or stage 4 pressure injury;
- Deep tissue injury is intact or nonintact skin with localized area of persistent non-blanchable deep red maroon, purple discoloration or epidermal separation revealing a dark wound bed or blood-filled blister;
- Medical device-related pressure injuries result from the use of devices designed and applied for diagnostic or therapeutic purposes and is staged using the staging system; and
- Mucous membrane pressure injuries are found on mucous membranes with a history of a medical device in use at the location of the injury.[13]

A valid risk assessment tool should be used to perform a risk assessment upon admission and periodically on a scheduled basis or when there are significant changes in condition. Intrinsic as well as extrinsic risk factors should be examined, and high-risk settings and groups should be targeted. Patients with immobility, who are at higher risk, should be monitored frequently. Assessment should also include differentiation from other types of wounds, any fecal or urinary incontinence, and subsequent management. Other factors that may impede healing should also be included such as tobacco use, nutritional assessment, support surfaces, previous treatments, prior ulcers, and surgical interventions.[14] Knowledge and research regarding pressure injuries continues to expand. Some of the recent literature based on Black and Gefen's research reported on the importance of managing the microclimate to prevent pressure injuries.[15] Treatment of pressure injuries also includes educating the patient and caregivers about preventive strategies, promoting healing, and preventing recurrences with the emphasis on lifelong changes.

Pressure, friction, and shear, known factors for pressure injury development, should be minimized or eliminated; this includes pressure from any medical devices. Elevating the heels, turning, repositioning, and offloading pressure from bony prominences are vital to treatment. If these issues are not addressed, the wound will continue to decline or not heal in spite of other treatments. The head of the bed should be at or below 30° or in the lowest elevation tolerable for the patient's medical condition to avoid shearing. Anyone mobility impaired, bedbound, or chairbound should be scheduled for regular repositioning and turning. Special attention should be paid to the anatomy, postural alignment, distribution of weight, and support of the feet with positioning.[14]

Support surfaces on beds and chairs should be used but do not eliminate the need for repositioning. The support surface for the bed and the chair should meet the patient's needs and be compatible with the care setting.[14] Algorithms such as the Wound, Ostomy, Continence Nurse (WOCN) Society's Evidence- and Consensus-Based Support Surface Algorithm can be used to identify appropriate surfaces (http://algorithm.wocn.org) for individuals aged 16 years or older and for bariatric patients.[14] Nixon, Smith, Brown, and colleagues'[15] study provided additional confirmation that high-specification foam mattresses are advised in high-risk patients and that alternating pressure mattresses should be considered when foam mattresses are not successful in prevention strategies. Foam rings, cutouts, and donut-type devices should be avoided due to increased pressure to the surrounding tissue.[14] Additionally, the investigators have experienced positive results in collaboration with physical therapist who specializes in wheelchair and seating for wheelchair seating and cushion evaluations, which include mapping to secure the most effective cushions for wheelchair-bound patients.

A significant part of the treatment involves examining the whole patient, which would include screening and managing nutritional deficits, and other medical conditions such as hydration, anemia, and diabetes. It is advised that a minimum of 30 to 35 kcal/kg body weight/d, 1.25 to 1.5 g of protein/kg body weight/d, and 1 mL of fluid intake/kcal/d is offered to individuals with nutritional and pressure injury risks.[14] Individualized bowel and bladder management should be instituted for those with incontinence.[14]

Skin barriers can be used as a preventive measure to protect and maintain skin integrity. Prophylactic dressings to the sacral and heel areas should be considered in at-risk patients, especially the bedbound. On open wounds, appropriate solutions should be selected for cleansing and the periwound area should be included with cleansing. The wound should be monitored and assessed with each dressing change to determine if the type of dressing is appropriate or needs modification. Preparing the wound bed includes debriding when there is a high suspicion of wound biofilm or when there is nonviable tissue present. Dressings to maintain moisture balance and eliminate dead space are advised. Antibiotics should be initiated based on clinical evidence and by determining the bacterial bioburden by tissue biopsy or Levine quantitative swab technique. A 2-week course of topical antibiotics should be considered for nonhealing pressure ulcers. However, if bacteremia, advancing cellulitis, sepsis, or osteomyelitis is present, systemic antibiotics and medical management will be needed. Antiseptics should be considered for wounds that are not expected to heal or for wounds that are critically colonized.[14]

There is evidence that adjunctive therapies can be beneficial and should be considered for pressure injuries. These therapies include platelet-derived growth factor, electrical stimulation, and negative pressure wound therapy as indicated. If stage 3 and 4 pressure injuries do not respond to conservative measures, then consideration should be given for operative repair. Appropriate screening for surgical candidates is needed to optimize the success and avoid postoperative complications. Pain control measures to eliminate or control the source of pain are also a part of the overall plan. It is also recognized that complete healing may not be realistic in some patients, and therefore plans for long-term management may be needed.[14]

CONSIDERATIONS
Wound Healing

The depth of skin injury determines the mechanism for wound repair. Shallow injuries involving the epidermal and superficial dermal layers heal by regeneration. However, injuries involving deep dermal structures, subcutaneous tissue, muscle, tendon, ligaments, and bone heal by scar formation because they are unable to regenerate.[1] Other factors to consider are if the wound is acute versus chronic and if the repair is primary, secondary, or tertiary.[1] Typically, acute wounds occur suddenly and may involve trauma or surgery and generally have a faster and stronger closure. Chronic wounds typically involve vascular issues, long-term inflammation, or injury that is repetitive to the tissue and have a longer healing course or may not heal.[1]

Primary, secondary, and tertiary wound healing is based on surgical concepts. In primary wound healing, the incisional wound edges are approximated surgically. Wound healing is faster and with less scar tissue as long as secondary complications such as infection are avoided. Secondary wound healing allows the wound to heal by scar formation because it is left open and is a slower process. Sometimes wounds have a delayed closure where the wound is cleaned of debris or the risk of infection is resolved before surgical closure; this is called *tertiary wound closure*.[1]

The process of wound healing is continuous and involves a series of stages. The process does not end with wound closure because remodeling of tissue may take up to 18 months after wound closure. In acute wounds, the cascade of healing involves 4 overlapping phases: hemostasis, inflammatory phase, proliferation phase, and maturation phase.[2]

- Hemostasis: clot formation occurs to control blood loss and provide a temporary bacterial barrier. The clot also has growth factors and provides a matrix for scaffolding of migrating cells.[1] This step is followed by breakdown of the clot wherein substances are released that attract cells needed to begin repair and provide fuel for the process.[1]
- Inflammation: the wound bed is cleaned, and the focus is on the control of infection. The complement system is activated, which lyses and destroys target cells and helps to bind neutrophils in bacteria, facilitating phagocytosis and bacterial destruction.[2] The 2 main inflammatory cells neutrophils and macrophages are a major part of the acute inflammatory process. There are multiple cytokines depending on the cell source that have specific biologic activity resulting in diverse effects on the wound healing process.[2]
- Proliferation: epithelialization, granulation tissue formation, neoangiogenesis, as well as matrix deposition and collagen synthesis. Many factors are involved including perfusion, oxygenation, nutritional status, and glucose levels.[1,2]

- Maturation or remodeling: begins around 3 weeks and continues past 1 year. The scar tissue formed is stiff and has less tensile strength than the original tissue. In addition, imbalances in synthesis and degradation of the matrix can result in complications such as hypertrophic scarring, keloid formation, or wound break-down. Hypoxia, malnutrition, and excess levels of MMPs are typically involved in wound breakdown at this phase.[1]

Because the average length of stay in an inpatient rehabilitation setting is approximately 13.8 days, it is clear why education for staff, patients, and care providers during and after rehabilitation is key for assessing, managing, and optimizing skin care; preventing wounds; and promoting wound healing. It is also clear why the overall health as well as the wound needs to be assessed and managed during this process.

Dressings

A proliferation of wound dressings occurred over the past 2 decades after empirical research provided evidence for moist wound healing. Moist wound healing has now been accepted by most clinicians as best practice. Selecting the most appropriate wound dressing can be quite daunting because more than 2000 products were noted on the market several years ago.[16,17]

The clinician should be knowledgeable of the wound care product's advantages, disadvantages, interactions, and contraindications before prescribing or using on a patient. In addition, the anatomic location of the wound, the available forms of the product, cost, ease of application, and access should all be considered. Some dressings serve multiple purposes. Neither do wound dressings follow the one-size-fits-all approach any more nor are the same dressings used throughout the healing process. The wound should be assessed at each dressing change to determine if the current wound dressing is most appropriate or if it should be changed.[16,17] Some of the principles of care to consider in selecting wound dressings are as follows:

- Identify patient goals and preferences
- Assess and collect data and address concerns about the patient's overall health
- Support the body's tissue defense system
- Use nontoxic wound cleansers
- Eliminate dead space (tunnels, tracts, and undermining)
- Maintain a moist wound bed environment/manage the drainage
- Remove nonviable tissue and infection
- Minimize trauma to the wound bed
- Protect the periwound area from trauma and infection
- Pain management[2,17]

SUMMARY

Some of the most common skin issues affecting individuals in rehabilitation settings are aging skin, incontinence dermatitis, intertrigo/yeast, surgical wounds, and pressure injuries. Pressure injuries can be some of the most devastating. The ultimate goal is to maintain skin integrity so that the skin can optimally function to provide protection, thermoregulation, sensation, metabolism, and communication. In all these skin issues, assessment, prevention, early intervention, management, and treatment using science-based strategies are advised.

CLINICS CARE POINTS

- Treat the whole person
- Perform consistent, thorough assessments to determine the cause and type of alteration in skin integrity
- Eliminate and/or minimize causative factors
- Assess wounds with each dressing change to determine the appropriate dressing.
- Educate patient and caregivers on preventive strategies and management
- Prevention and/or early intervention are goals to optimize skin management
- Some chronic wounds are not expected to heal.

DISCLOSURES

The authors have nothing to disclose.

REFERENCES

1. Bryant R, Nix D. Acute & chronic wounds current management concepts. 5th Edition. St. Louis: Elsevier; 2016.
2. Baranoski S, Ayello E. Wound care essentials practice principles. 5th Edition. Philadelphia: Lippincott Williams & Wilkins; 2020.
3. Jacelon CS. The specialty practice of rehabilitation nursing, a core curriculum. In: Anderson C, Kautz D, et al, editors. Chapter 7 physical healthcare patterns and nursing interventions. 6th Edition. Glenview (IL): Association of Rehabilitation Nurses; 2011. p. 109–11.
4. Dyer JM, Miller RA. Chronic skin fragility of aging: current concepts in the pathogenesis, recognition, and management of dermatoporosis. J Clin Aesthet Dermatol 2018;11(1):13–8.
5. Russell-Goldman E, Murphy G. July2020, american journal of pathology, the pathobiology of skin aging. Am J Pathol 2020;190:1356e1369. https://doi.org/10.1016/j.ajpath.2020.03.007.
6. Gray M, Bliss DZ, Doughty DB, et al. Incontinence-associated dermatitis: a consensus. J Wound Ostomy Continence Nurs 2007;34:45–54.
7. Zulkowski K. Understanding Moisture-Associated Skin Damage, Medical Adhesive-Related Skin Injuries, and Skin Tears. Adv Skin Wound Care 2017 Aug;30(8):372–81.
8. Black J, Gray M, Bliss D, et al. MASD Part 2: incontinence-associated dermatitis and intertriginous dermatitis. A consensus. J Wound Ostomy Continence Nurs 2011;38(4):359–70. Lippincott, Williams, & Wilkins.
9. Gray M, Beeckman D, Bliss D, et al. Incontinence-associated dermatitis: a comprehensive review and update. J Wound Ostomy Continence Nurs 2012; 39(1):61–74. Lippincott, Williams & Wilkins.
10. Beeckman D, Campbell J, Campbell K, et al. Proceedings of the Global IAD Expert Panel. Incontinence associated dermatitis: moving prevention forward. London SE1 9PG, UK: Wounds International; 2015. Available at: www.woundsinternational.com. Accessed February 26, 2021.
11. Berríos-Torres SI, Umscheid CA, Bratzler DW, et al. Centers for disease control and prevention guideline for the prevention of surgical site infection, 2017. JAMA Surg 2017;152(8):784–91.

12. Sprigle S, McNair D, Sonenblum S. Pressure ulcer risk factors in persons with mobility-related disabilities. Adv Skin Wound Care 2020;33:148–54.

13. Edsberg LE, Black JM, Goldberg M, et al. Sieggreen, Mary revised national pressure ulcer advisory panel pressure injury staging system. J Wound Ostomy Continence Nurs 2016;43(6):585–97.

14. Wound, ostomy and continence nurses society-wound guidelines task force WOCN 2016 guideline for prevention and management of pressure injuries (Ulcers). J Wound Ostomy Continence Nurs 2017;44(3):241–6. https://doi.org/10.1097/WON.0000000000000321.

15. Saindon K, Berlowitz D. Update on pressure injuries: a review of the literature. Adv Skin Wound Care 2020;33:403–9.

16. Hess C. CWOCN quick tips: choosing a wound dressing. Adv Skin Wound Care 2005;18(2):70–2.

17. Baranoski S, Ayello EA. Wound dressings: an evolving art and science. Adv Skin Wound Care 2012;25(2):87–92 [Quiz: 92-4].

Considerations for Skin and Wound Care in Pediatric Patients

Elizabeth Day Dechant, BSN, RN, CWOCN, CFCN

KEYWORDS

- Pediatric • Wound • Skin • Neonate

KEY POINTS

- Pediatric wound care is a subspecialty field that requires a collaborative and holistic approach to meet the goals of all members of the care team as well as the needs of the patient and their family.
- Pediatric patients range from birth to late teens and may have a wide variety of wound types that should be treated using evidence-based principles with consideration of the neurodevelopmental stage of the child and available resources.
- Children have unique risk factors that predispose them to iatrogenic skin injuries.
- Children with neuromuscular conditions and dependence on medical devices are challenged with chronic skin issues.
- Certified wound, ostomy, continence nurses are needed as wound care experts to help to develop evidence-based skin care regimens and updated wound treatment practices. They are also in a prime role to facilitate communication and collaboration among providers to stimulate and support progress and additional research in pediatric wound care.

INTRODUCTION

Wound care practices continue to evolve as we learn more about the physiology of wound healing as well as factors that lead to wound recalcitrance. Wound care in pediatrics is a subspecialty field guided by limited literature. Many of the available articles on pediatric skin and wound-related topics make note of the sparse evidence and point to the need for additional research to guide standardization of care.[1–4]

Despite an ever-increasing array of product choices, pediatric skin care and wound treatment protocols are often the result of individual preference[1–3] or availability of products within an institution. It is generally assumed that wounds in children heal quickly and without complications,[1–3] making the topic of wound care and nonhealing wounds in pediatrics of less interest.[3] In the absence of experts to guide practice, treatments are frequently outdated and include broad use of antiquated methods

The author has nothing to disclose.
Children's of Alabama, 1600 7th Avenue South, Birmingham, AL 35233, USA
E-mail address: elizabeth.dechant@childrensal.org

Phys Med Rehabil Clin N Am 33 (2022) 759–771
https://doi.org/10.1016/j.pmr.2022.06.009

such as wet-to-dry dressings.[1,2,5] Lack of research on the use of advanced wound care products in pediatric patients leaves clinicians without sufficient evidence to support their treatment decisions.[1-4]

The availability of providers specializing in pediatric wound care is very limited. Certified wound ostomy continence (WOC) nurses have specialized training with expertise in skin, wound, and ostomy care.[6] Experts are needed to evaluate the available literature and formulate best practice guidelines with consideration for products and methods that best meet the complex needs of pediatric patients and their caregivers.[1-4]

AGE-RELATED CONSIDERATIONS

The term "pediatric" encompasses patients from birth to late teens, which presents a wide range of physiologic and neurodevelopmental considerations.

Preemies and Neonates

More and more babies are surviving prematurity as early as 22 to 23 weeks gestation. In fact, the world's most premature baby had his first birthday in June 2021. He was born at 21 weeks and 2 days gestation.[7]

Increased risk for skin damage in neonates is well-documented, with even higher risk in preemies. Some issues to consider are as follows:

- Very thin or absent stratum corneum in premature neonates results in compromised barrier function and increased infection risk, as well as impaired thermoregulation and a higher rate of transepidermal water loss and electrolyte imbalance.[1,2,8,9]
- Thinner, more permeable skin, compounded by increased body surface area to weight ratio means preemies and neonates are more susceptible to adverse effects due to percutaneous absorption of irritants (alcohol, betadine, and so forth).[1,2,8,9]
- An immature dermoepidermal junction makes neonates more prone to skin stripping and tension blisters secondary to use of medical adhesives.[1,2,8,9]

The fundamental goal of care in most neonatal wounds should be to gently support their naturally brisk healing process while preventing pain and secondary injury. Advanced wound-care products should be selected to minimize pain and frequency of dressing changes.[1,2,4,8,9] A general recommendation is to avoid the use of any potentially absorbable topical agents on the skin before 1 month of age,[4] although consideration of a product's risk versus benefit should be made. Adhesives for neonatal wound care should be limited to silicone-based dressings and tapes,[1,2,4,8,9] and avoided altogether when possible, opting instead for soft stretchy tubular bandages or wraps to secure dressings.[2,9] Liquid skin barrier films and adhesive removal agents that are silicone-based and alcohol-free, do not leave a residue and should be used to mitigate medical adhesive-related skin injury (MARSI).[9]

Infants and Toddlers

As babies get older, they may become more active, curious, and mobile. Maintaining a clean, occlusive wound dressing is challenging in infants who may begin to pull off dressings or in children who are crawling, running, or playing.[1] It may be necessary to secure medical devices with soft restraints, elastic wraps, or specially designed belts or vests.[10]

Adolescents and Teenagers

Older children present with mixed issues based on their developmental stage and the type of wound care needed. Anxiety or fear may be based on the "unknown" even if wound care is not necessarily painful. Body-image concerns may relate to lack of privacy or potential for scarring.[9] All of these factors should be patiently assessed and discussed with patients and their caregivers, allowing the child as much autonomy and decision-making as possible.

PAIN, FEAR, AND ANXIETY

Children experience and express pain, fear, and anxiety differently than adults.[4] Caregivers may also be anxious about their child's condition or learning to provide wound care.

Management of these issues is a priority. Each step of a dressing change should be explained to the patient, and they should be warned if something may be cold or may cause pain. If feasible, children should be allowed to call a "time out" when they need a break during the procedure. Children may participate in their own wound care as is developmentally appropriate.[2,4] This builds trust and gives the child the feeling that they have some control over the process. Primary caregivers should be involved to provide support and distraction. If possible, parents may hold, cuddle, or feed their infants or smaller children to comfort them during dressing changes.[2,4] Child life specialists[4] are specially trained professionals who help children of all ages understand and cope with medical care. Allowing children to play video games or watch television during wound care is another option for distraction. Management of pain may include premedication with oral or IV medications[2,4] or the use of topical anesthetics such as lidocaine gel.[11] Use of polymeric membrane dressings has been proven to reduce pain.[12] Procedural sedation or even general anesthesia is sometimes required for complex procedures. Nitrous gas has been shown to be beneficial because it effectively reduces anxiety and wears off quickly.[4]

An added source of stress, confusion, and mistrust for parents is the frequent discrepancy in wound care recommendations among providers.[9] A lack of wound care knowledge has been reported as the primary barrier to optimal wound management among hospitalists[13] and surgical specialists continue to prefer outdated wound care methods such as wet-to-dry dressings[5] that are no longer evidence-based.[1,2,5,14]

WOUND HEALING IN CHILDREN

Wounds in neonates and children follow the same physiological pathway to healing as in adults.[4] This is a dynamic process that follows a predictable series of overlapping phases, which includes an inflammatory phase, a proliferative phase, and a remodeling/maturation phase.[1,4] The goals of wound care that underlie the treatment of all wounds, regardless of patient age include identification and treatment of infection, debridement of nonviable tissue, maintenance of a clean, moist wound bed with absorption of exudate, and protection of the wound to prevent secondary skin breakdown or infection.[1]

Due to faster rates of cell proliferation and collagen production, as well as increased amounts of fibroblasts, pediatric wounds typically heal more quickly than wounds in adults.[2,4,8] Factors that may complicate wound healing include malnutrition, medications (vasopressors, steroids), infection, limited mobility,[2,4] and socioeconomic status.[4] Even in uncomplicated cases, it is beneficial to select advanced dressings[9] and treatment methods that support the aforementioned goals of care[1] and also:

- Address the needs of the whole patient and their family.[4,9] This includes factors such as age, developmental stage of the child, the child's overall condition and accompanying issues and the availability of competent caregivers. Insurance coverage for supplies, as well as transportation issues and lack of resources may limit care options.
- Consider the physiologic needs of immature skin, including propensity for skin stripping and increased absorption of topical agents.[1,2,4,8,9]
- Minimize the patient's pain, fear, and anxiety.[1,2,4,9] Concerns of parents and caregivers must also be considered.[2,4,9]
- Are relatively simple and easily understood.[9]
- Are cost-effective.

WOUND TYPES IN CHILDREN

Causes of wounds in pediatric patients range from congenital conditions and disease processes to surgery, trauma, and iatrogenic injuries.[1,2,4,9]

Wounds secondary to congenital or acquired disease processes may be acute (eg, perfusion injuries, staphylococcal scalded skin syndrome, Stevens-Johnson syndrome) or chronic (eg, atopic dermatitis, epidermolysis bullosa, hidradenitis suppurativa) and are most effectively treated through careful collaboration and ongoing assessment by primary care providers, specialists, WOC nurses, and the patient's caregivers.

Medical and surgical advances have led to increased survivability of complex conditions.[1] Hospitalized children, as well as children with neuromuscular disorders or other medically fragile conditions are at risk for acute or recurrent skin breakdown due to moisture, pressure, friction, and medical devices. Iatrogenic skin injuries include pressure injuries (PIs), moisture-associated skin damage (MASD), extravasation injuries, MARSI, and irritant or contact-associated dermatitis. Chronically ill children may be frequently hospitalized and have intrinsic factors that predispose them for recurrent skin issues and poor wound healing.[1]

Pressure Injuries

Historically associated with the geriatric population, hospital-acquired PIs (HAPIs) are one of the most common "never events" among pediatric patients.[3] Rates are highest among older (larger) children and in critical care areas and pediatric rehab units. Occurrence is lowest in neonates and in general pediatric units.[3,15] The most severe PIs among pediatric patients occur in chronically ill children aged more than 8 years.[15] Higher acuity, immobility, cognitive and/or functional impairment, and extremes in BMI are also predictors of PI risk.[16]

Medical devices are the most common cause, accounting for up to 90% of pediatric HAPIs.[3] Respiratory devices are at the top of the list of devices causing skin injury.[3,16] Immobilizers, gastric tubes, and external monitoring devices are next in the list of devices causing skin injury.[16]

Pediatric patients have a unique and different set of risk factors for development of PIs than adult patients:

- Pediatric patients range from micropreemies to adult-sized teenagers, making it difficult to find medical devices that fit all size needs. Most devices are scaled-down versions of adult devices, not designed with consideration of pediatric risk factors. Ill-fitting devices are more likely to cause injuries.[3,16]
- A wide range of patient sizes also makes it difficult to create standard PI prevention guidelines that meet the needs of all pediatric patients.[3]

- Differences in body weight distribution influence the location of immobility-related PIs. The occiput is a common site for PIs in infants and children aged younger than 5 years.[3]
- A higher ratio of adipose tissue to muscle and softer tissue structure in younger children creates increased tissue deformability.[3]
- Children often require additional securement of devices because they may not understand the necessity of the device and may try to remove it.[16]
- Babies and young children lack the ability to communicate pain specific to PI development or medical devices that may be too tight.[3]

PI risk assessment tools are a good starting point toward prevention but often fall short.[3] Risk factors that are not assessed by any of the scales include dark skin tone and the presence of thick or dark hair in infants and children. These factors may obscure early detection of PIs, particularly on the occiput.

Critical points in PI prevention include frequent repositioning and thorough skin inspection, including all skin folds and skin under removable medical devices. Medical devices should be frequently repositioned as possible and padded with appropriate dressings,[16] most commonly foam.[1,3] Use of appropriate support surfaces is paramount.[3] Fluidized positioners offer customization of pressure redistribution for immobile patients because they can be molded around body contours and can help offload pressure from cords and tubing. The use of positioning aids such as rolled linens should be strictly avoided because this can quickly lead to PIs.

Incontinence-Associated Dermatitis and moisture-associated skin damage

Incontinence-associated dermatitis (IAD), a.k.a. diaper rash, is one of the most common skin problems seen in pediatric patients.[1,2,4,17] IAD affects healthy children who are not yet potty-trained as well as children of all ages with bowel and bladder incontinence.[17] Chronic IAD can be a source of extreme stress for parents.

IAD occurs when excess moisture and increased pH from stool and urine cause breakdown of the natural acidic barrier function of the skin. Skin becomes macerated and is more permeable to microorganisms and more susceptible to damage by fecal enzymes, friction, and pressure.[4,9,17]

Prevention of IAD is key. Chronic impairment of skin barrier function has been noted in patients with recurrent IAD.[17] Preventative care includes maintenance of dry, acidic skin (pH 4–6). Wipes and cleansers should be alcohol-free, fragrance-free, and pH neutral. Disposable diapers are preferred for their breathable cover and superabsorbent core that pulls moisture away from the skin. Diapers should be changed frequently. Routine use of liquid barrier films, creams, or ointments that are silicone or petrolatum-based may help prevent IAD.[9,17]

When IAD occurs, a thick layer of barrier cream containing ingredients such as zinc, petrolatum, or carboxymethylcellulose should be maintained on the skin to promote healing and provide a barrier to stool and urine. With each diaper change, the skin should be wiped very gently, avoiding removal of all products, and more barrier cream should be applied.[9,17]

If skin is denuded, "crusting" is a very effective method to promote healing and provide a more durable skin barrier. To "crust" the skin, a pectin-based powder (stoma powder) is sprinkled on denuded areas and then sealed with a silicone-based, alcohol-free liquid skin barrier film.[1,3,9] These layers may be repeated 1 to 2 more times before applying a thick layer of zinc-based barrier cream. This "crust" will wear off as the skin heals and should not be removed prematurely. Crusting should be repeated as needed when all layers of products have worn off the skin or after bathing. "Airing out" denuded skin is a common myth and should be avoided.[9]

Persistent IAD that is not responding to crusting may require a more durable skin barrier. Cyanoacrylate skin barrier film (Marathon, Medline) is very effective in healing stubborn IAD as well as MASD as around enterostomies or percutaneous tubes.[1]

Fungal dermatitis can be recognized by its distinct, erythematous maculopapular rash with satellite lesions that often covers a larger area of skin including the inguinal folds. This should be treated with a topical antifungal. If the skin is also denuded, antifungals should be layered under a zinc-based barrier cream. Antifungal powder may also be applied in conjunction with a silicone-based, alcohol-free liquid skin barrier film using the "crusting" method described above, before applying a thick layer of barrier cream.[9]

Prevention and management strategies for IAD should also be extended to other forms of MASD, which may occur around various percutaneous drains, tubes, and ostomies, as well as in skin folds or under medical devices. Use of the crusting technique or cyanoacrylates should be considered[1] in addition to the use of absorbent foam dressings, moisture-wicking fabrics[18] and hydroconductive dressings (Beier Drawtex Healthcare, South Africa). Management of MASD around a tracheostomy should be limited to the use of absorbent dressings (foams, hydroconductive) only. Moisture-retentive dressings as well as ointments and powders should be avoided around the trach stoma.[9]

Extravasation Injuries

Hospitalized children often require long-term use of intravenous lines to provide medications and nutrition. The tendency to tape and wrap intravenous lines in children may preclude frequent assessment and early detection of extravasation, leading to extensive tissue damage.[19]

Prevention of extravasation injuries should focus on close monitoring of peripheral venous lines and the use of central venous catheters whenever possible. When an extravasation occurs and visible discoloration or bulla formation is noted, hyaluronidase should be administered subcutaneously around the site to reduce local tissue damage. For extravasation of vasoconstrictors, phentolamine is the antidote of choice. If the injury is limited to edema, it is often well-managed with the elevation of the extremity and frequent monitoring of distal perfusion. The use of heat or cold is no longer recommended. Principles of moist wound healing should be initiated early to prevent progression of tissue damage and eschar formation.[9]

Enterostomy Tubes

Enteral feeding tubes are a very common device used in pediatric patients to administer nutrition, fluids, and medications. They may also be used for decompression of the stomach and GI tract. These include nasogastric or orogastric tubes as well as surgically placed gastrostomy tubes, gastrojejunostomy tubes, or jejunostomy tubes.[10]

In patients with long-term percutaneous gastrostomy tubes, complications are common, with skin problems being one of the most frequent issues. Hypergranulation tissue, site infection, leakage from the stoma and resultant irritant dermatitis often occur.[10,20,21] These relatively minor complications also lead to many unanticipated ED and clinic visits that could be mitigated through caregiver education and readily available clinicians to handle issues via phone or email.[22]

The prevention of peristomal complications is best achieved with a consistent skin care regimen and stabilization of the tube because excess movement leads to erosion of the stoma, leakage, and subsequent skin complications. Extension tubing should be removed when not in use and should be secured to the abdomen when connected.[10] Meticulous stabilization is particularly important in the postoperative period to help establish a secure tract around the tube so that complications are minimized.[21] Peristomal irritant dermatitis is treated with a variety of methods including barrier products, crusting, and the use of absorbent dressings[10,20] (eg, foam, gauze, cloth, hydroconductive). Best practices for the treatment of hypergranulation tissue are debated, with options including salt-based products, steroid creams, cauterization with silver nitrate and surgical excision.[9,10,20] More important than the topical treatment choice, which can vary widely, is thoroughly educating parents and caregivers about realistic expectations and empowering them with the knowledge and resources to handle minor complications.[22]

Neuromuscular Conditions

There are multiple pediatric neuromuscular diagnoses, which share common complications resulting primarily from immobility and weakness. Examples include cerebral palsy, myelomeningocele (spina bifida), and acquired brain or spinal cord injuries.[23] Although this population of patients may be more frequently hospitalized, they are primarily managed at home and present a range of skin-related challenges for their caregivers.

- Physical deformities create difficulties with positioning and upright seating.[23] Offloading pressure from bony prominences may be challenging because offloading one "high-risk" area often increases pressure on another.
- Severe scoliosis and joint contractures may result in deep skin folds that have a propensity for increased moisture and friction, resulting in intertriginous dermatitis.
- Limited motor function for performing self-care activities and reduced mobility and sensation[23] puts patients at risk for developing PIs and IAD or MASD.
- Gastrointestinal complications include malnutrition and obesity,[23] which lead to decreased tissue integrity and a higher propensity for skin damage.

Caregivers must be diligent with frequent skin assessments to proactively detect and manage these issues. Basic maintenance of healthy skin integrity starts with topical cleansers and products that support low skin pH (4–6).[17] Moisture-wicking fabrics,[18] thin foam dressings, and transparent barrier products are good choices for problematic skin folds. PIs are avoided with routine repositioning and offloading of problem areas and ensuring that support surfaces and assistive devices are appropriate.[3] Children who require long-term medical devices such as orthopedic splints and braces or specialty seating should be routinely reevaluated because they grow to ensure appropriate fit and function as well as to prevent skin injuries.

WOUND DRESSING SELECTION

Topical wound care products should be chosen according to their moisture-retentive or absorptive properties and current goals of wound care based on the phase of healing and other needs of the patient.[1,4,8,9] A general guideline for all pediatric wounds is to select a dressing that is secure and durable but does not impede the child's movement or activity, is atraumatic and painless on removal, and allows maximum time between dressing changes.[1,8,9] Advanced wound dressings should be considered as first-line treatments to achieve these goals.[1,9] The use of foams, hydrogels, hydrocolloids, skin barriers, and silicone-based products has been widely documented in pediatric wound care.[1,2,4,8] Additional product choices are listed in the Pediatric Wound Care Toolkit (**Fig. 1**) and have varying amounts of evidence to describe their use. A complete "toolkit" supports a customized wound care treatment plan to meet the individual needs of each patient. Treatment choices may be limited by institutional product formularies and insurance coverage, requiring exploration of alternative resources such as community-based agencies and even charitable organizations.

Wound Cleansing

Water and normal saline are the cleansers of choice for pediatric wounds.[2] Wounds that are clean and granulating or epithelializing do not necessarily require cleaning with every dressing change.[4] Hypochlorous acid is a noncytotoxic, antimicrobial wound and skin cleanser that is extremely safe and gentle for children of all ages, even on mucous membranes. It has no clinical contraindications in children.[24] Ideally, cleansers should be warmed to body temperature.[2,4]

Choices for Debridement

Autolytic debridement is the most common debridement method used in pediatric wound care.[4] It is gentle and safe, using the body's own enzymes and fluids to selectively eliminate nonviable tissue from wounds. Autolytic debridement is supported by a variety of moist dressings and extended time between dressing changes.[14] Some examples of products that promote autolytic debridement are dressings and gels containing leptospermum honey, moisture-donating wound gels and zinc-based hydrophilic paste (Triad, Coloplast, Mankato, MN). I have found the zinc-based hydrophilic dressing to be the most versatile because it is also an effective moisture barrier and can be used without a cover dressing on wounds in the diaper area or on other areas of the body, where maintaining a dressing can be very difficult.

Options for chemical debridement of nonviable tissue include the use of solutions or gels containing sodium hypochlorite[14] or hypochlorous acid.[24] Although sodium hypochlorite has been deemed cytotoxic even in low concentrations (>0.0005%), hypochlorous acid is safe for use during all stages of healing.[24]

Enzymatic debridement uses collagenase (Santyl, Smith & Nephew, Fort Worth , TX) ointment to selectively separate nonviable tissue from a wound bed. It has been well-studied and is a standard tool in the care of adult wounds.[14] There are only a few articles documenting its use in pediatric patients but all of them note that collagenase has been found to be safe and effective in children, including neonates.[25]

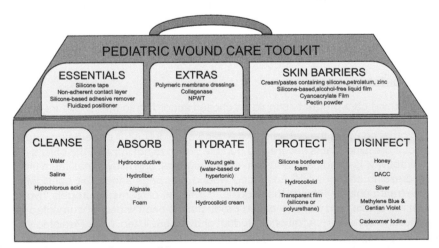

Fig. 1. Pediatric wound care toolkit.

Selective sharp or surgical debridement may be indicated for larger wounds with increased amounts of nonviable tissue.[4] As discussed in "Negative Pressure Wound Therapy" section, negative pressure wound therapy with instillation may be an ideal alternative for debridement of larger wounds to prevent recurrent OR trips.[26]

Treating Infection

The need for and use of topical antimicrobial products in pediatric wound care continues to be explored. Although prophylactic use of systemic antibiotics is discouraged,[4,27] broad spectrum topical antimicrobials may be beneficial in treating wounds with signs of critical colonization that may be impeding wound healing.[1,27] Ideal choices include hypochlorous acid,[10,24] and products or dressings that contain leptospermum honey, ionic or nanocrystalline silver,[1,4,27] or a combination of methylene blue and gentian violet.[27] Dialkylcarbamoyl chloride-coated dressings physically bind and remove bacteria.[27] Although limited evidence in pediatric wounds exists, cadexomer iodine has been proven as the only topical product to effectively treat bacterial biofilm,[28] so its benefit versus risk in children must be weighed by experienced wound care providers.

Polymeric Membrane Dressings

Polymeric membrane dressings (PMDs, PolyMem, Ferris Mfg. Group, Fort Worth, TX) represent a unique category of dressings that are innovative and multifunctional.[12] PMDs meet many of the wound care needs in the pediatric population and have been proven safe in extremely premature neonates.[29] PMDs are often categorized with other foam dressings but this assumption overlooks the many benefits that set them apart. Invented to treat pediatric burns, they are designed to support healing in all phases and prevent adhesion to the wound bed. PMDs are made of a flexible hydrophilic membrane and an absorbent core containing ingredients, which provide continuous cleaning and support autolysis. PMDs reduce inflammation and edema, even on closed injuries such as bruises and hematomas. They are the only drug-free dressing shown to reduce pain. They are easily conformable and do not require frequent dressing changes,[12] making them ideal for a wide range of pediatric wound types, from minor skin lesions to complex chronic conditions such as epidermolysis bullosa.[12] **Fig. 2** shows gastrostomy tube site with a stage 3 PI and denuded irritant dermatitis successfully treated with a PMD.

Negative Pressure Wound Therapy

Negative pressure wound therapy (NPWT) is an "active" therapy that supports healing of larger or more complex wounds using reticulated foam placed in the wound bed and connected to a pump that provides negative pressure to stimulate perfusion and granulation tissue formation on a microscopic level while controlling exudate

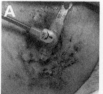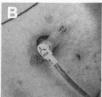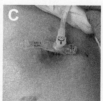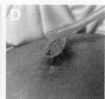

Fig. 2. (*A*) Day 0. (*B*) Day 8. (*C*) Day 10. (*D*) Day 13. Site treated with polymeric membrane dressing changed as needed when soiled.

and tissue edema on a macroscopic level. NPWT provides an occlusive dressing that reduces bioburden and secondary contamination. It requires less frequent dressing changes, usually 2 to 3 times per week and is not likely to be removed by the patient. NPWT is used on a variety of open and closed surgical wounds, traumatic wounds, and PIs. It has proven to be safe in children of all ages.[1,2,8,9]

For larger wounds with increased amounts nonviable tissue in the wound bed, NPWT with instillation and dwell (NPWTi-d) offers the option to introduce saline or other surfactant solutions into the wound bed at a specified frequency and dwell time to potentially reduce the need for surgical debridement.[26] **Fig. 3** shows a large wound successfully treated with NPWTi-d to help an 11-year-old patient with type I diabetes avoid repeat operating room (OR) trips.

Several factors should be considered when using NPWT in the pediatric population:

- The level of negative pressure should be kept near or below the child's mean arterial pressure to avoid any adverse effects.[1,8,9] Pressure should be started at lower levels and gradually increased. In older pediatric patients, guidelines for NPWT use are the same as those for adults.[9]
- NPWT dressing changes are typically more involved than a standard dressing change. Methods to reduce pain and provide distraction should be considered during all stages of the dressing change and during active therapy.
- Adhesive remover should be used to reduce pain during the removal of the dressing. NPWT drapes with silicone-based adhesive are more recently available and may be particularly beneficial to pediatric patients.

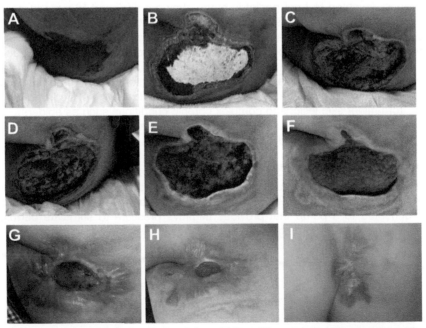

Fig. 3. (*A*) Day 0, deep tissue pressure injury (*B*) Day 30, autolytic debridement with zinc based cream. (*C*) Day 38, 2 days post surgical debridement. (*D*) Day 45, first NPWTi d dressing change (initiated on day 43). (*E*) Day 64, NPWTi d discontinued. (*F*) Day 82, treating with hydrofiber and hydroconductive dressings; pt. discharged 5 days later on day 87. (*G*) Day 159. (*H*) Day 178. (*I*) 3 months post healing. Complete healing was noted on Day 210.

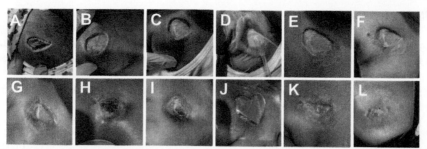

Fig. 4. (*A*) Day 0, necrosis at port site. (*B*) Day 11, s/p port removal. (*C*) Day 42, wound not heal-ing. (*D*) Day 42, NPWT initiated. (*E*) Day 46, first NPWT dressing change. (*F*) Day 49. (*G*) Day 63. (*H*) Day 70. (*I*) Day 84. (*J*) Day 84, discontinuation of NPWT, initiation of antimicrobial foam dressing. (*K*) Day 89. (*L*) Day 102, complete healing (60 days after placement of NPWT).

- Minimizing pain and bleeding during removal of foam from the wound bed can be accomplished through the use of a nonadherent contact layer under the foam. This also speeds dressing changes.[9]
- Periwound skin should be protected with a layer of transparent film or thin hydro-colloid dressing. An alcohol-free, silicone-based barrier film applied to the peri-wound skin reduces MASD and MARSI.[9]
- Use of the continuous, rather than intermittent, pressure setting is recommended to reduce pain during therapy because the intermittent pressure might be expe-rienced as pain or may be startling.[8,9]
- Use of a mechanical, rather than electric, pump for NPWT offers a more portable option for pediatric patients (SNAP Therapy System, KCI USA Inc., San Antonio, TX). The mechanical pump is about the size of a cell phone and can be worn on a small strap. The dressing is waterproof and is easily managed by caregivers. Dressing changes are done in an outpatient setting 2 to 3 times weekly. **Fig. 4** shows the rapid healing of a surgical site using a mechanical NPWT device on an 18-month-old with immune suppression.

SUMMARY
A Team-Based Approach

Provision of wound care to pediatric patients, whether on an inpatient or outpatient ba-sis, requires a collaborative approach.[6,9] In the hospital, care may be managed by a multidisciplinary team and involve subspecialties such as infectious disease, orthope-dics, gastroenterology, neurosurgery, and general or plastic surgery. Physical and occupational therapists, child life specialists, social workers, nurse case managers, child abuse specialists, and WOC nurses may also contribute to the patient's care. Con-flicting plans of care and gaps in communication or patient follow-up can have a nega-tive effect on patient outcomes.[9] Employment of WOC nurses to coordinate a plan for wound care has a positive effect on both patient outcomes and caregiver satisfaction.[7] It is the responsibility of the WOC nurse to facilitate communication and collaboration among all members of the care team, with a holistic consideration of the family's needs and resources to come up with a unified plan that meets everyone's goals.[7,9] Pediatric WOC nurses are tasked with pushing the boundaries of wound care practices by using their "toolkits" in often creative and innovative ways. This ultimately adds to the broader understanding and advancement of pediatric wound care practices through peer networking, education, and publication of case studies and other research.

CLINICS CARE POINTS

- Patiently addressing the patient's pain, fear, and anxiety regarding wound care as well as concerns of the caregiver is a priority.
- Select dressings with gentle, silicone-based adhesives, and advanced wound care products that allow extended time between dressing changes.
- Ensure medical devices fit appropriately and use appropriate dressings to mitigate pressure and moisture under/around devices.
- Frequent and thorough skin assessment is paramount in early detection and mitigation of many skin problems.

REFERENCES

1. King A, Stellar JJ, Blevins A, et al. Dressings and products in pediatric wound care. Adv Wound Care 2014;3(4):324–34.
2. Baharestani MM. An Overview of neonatal and pediatric wound care knowledge and considerations. Ostomy Wound Manage 2007;53(6):34–55.
3. Delmore B, Deppish M, Luna-Anderson C, et al. Pressure injuries in the pediatric population: a national pressure ulcer advisory panel white paper. Adv Skin Wound Care 2019;32(9):394–408.
4. Best Practice Statement. Principles of wound management in paediatric patients. London: Wounds UK; 2014.
5. Cowan LJ, Stechmiller J. Prevalence of wet-to-dry dressings in wound care. Adv Skin Wound Care 2009;22(12):567–73.
6. Wound, Ostomy and Continence Nurses Society Task Force. Wound, Ostomy, and Continence Nursing: Scope and Standards of WOC Practice, 2nd Edition: An Executive Summary. J Wound Ostomy Continence Nurs 2018;45(4):369–87.
7. Milward A. World's most premature baby, given 0% odds of survival, celebrates first birthday. Guinness Book of World Records website. Available at: https://www.guinnessworldrecords.com/news/2021/6/worlds-most-premature-baby-given-0-odds-of-survival-celebrates-first-birthday-663394. Accessed 8/17/2021.
8. Steen EH, WangX, Boochoon KS, et al. Wound healing and wound care in neonates: current therapies and novel options. Adv Skin Wound Care 2020;33(6):294–300.
9. Lund C, Singh C. Skin and wound care for neonatal and pediatric populations. In: Doughty DB, McNichol LL, editors. Wound, ostomy and continence nurses society core curriculum wound management. Philadelphia: Wolters Kluwer; 2016. p. p198–219.
10. Thompson NM. Nursing care and management of the gastrostomy and gastrojejunostomy tubes in the pediatric population. J Pediatr Surg Nurs 2019;8(4):97–111.
11. Agrawal V, Wilson K, Reyna R, et al. Feasibility of 4% topical lidocaine for pain management during negative pressure wound therapy dressing changes in pediatric patients. J Wound Ostomy Continence Nurs 2015;42(6):640–2.
12. Benskin LL. Evidence for polymeric membrane dressings as a unique dressing subcategory, using pressure ulcers as an example. Adv Wound Care 2018;7(12):419–26.
13. Walker CA, Rahman A, Gipson-Jones TL, et al. Hospitalists' needs assessment and perceived barriers in wound care management. J Wound Ostomy Continence Nurs 2019;46(2):98–105.

14. Ramundo JM. Principles and guidelines for wound debridement. In: Doughty DB, McNichol LL, editors. Wound, ostomy and continence nurses society core curriculum wound management. Philadelphia: Wolters Kluwer; 2016. p. p145–55.
15. Razmus I, Bergquist-Beringer S. Pressure injury prevalence and the rate of hospital-acquired pressure injury among pediatric patients in acute care. J Wound Ostomy Continence Nurs 2017;44(2):110–7.
16. Stellar JJ, Hasbani NR, Kulik LA, et al. Medical device-related pressure injuries in infants and children. J Wound Ostomy Continence Nurs 2020;47(5):459–69.
17. Lim YSL, Carville K. Prevention and management of incontinence-associated dermatitis in the pediatric population: an integrative review. J Wound Ostomy Continence Nurs 2019;46(1):30–7.
18. Singh C. Use of a moisture wicking fabric for prevention of skin damage around drains and parenteral access lines. J Wound Ostomy Continence Nurs 2016; 43(5):551–3.
19. McCullen KL, Pieper BA. Retrospective chart review of risk factors for extravasation among neonates receiving peripheral intravascular fluids. J Wound Ostomy Continence Nurs 2006;33(2):133–9.
20. Townley A, Wincentak J, Krog K, et al. Paediatric gastrostomy stoma complications and treatments: a rapid scoping review. J Clin Nurs 2018;27(7–8):1369–80.
21. Steen EH, Tuley JM, Balaji S, et al. The Use of a fixation dressing to reduce complications after neonatal gastrostomy tube Placement. Adv Wound Care 2020; 9(5):211–8.
22. Berman L, Hronek C, Raval MV, et al. Pediatric gastrostomy tube placement: lessons learned from high-performing institutions through structured interviews. Pediatr Qual Saf 2017;2(2):e01.
23. Skalsky AJ, Dalal PB. Common complications of pediatric neuromuscular disorders. Phys Med Rehabil Clin N Am 2015;26:21–8.
24. Couch K.S., Miller C., Cnossen L.A., et al., Non-cytotoxic wound bed preparation: Vashe hypochlorous acid wound cleansing solution. Wound Source White Paper. Available at: www.woundsource.com/sites/default/files/whitepapers/non-cytotoxic_wound_bed_preparation_white_paper.pdf. Accessed August 30, 2021.
25. Huett E, Bartley W, Morris D, et al. Collagenase for wound debridement in the neonatal intensive care unit: a retrospective case series. Pediatr Dermatol 2017;34(3):277–81.
26. Faust E, Opoku-Agyeman JL, Behnam AB. Use of negative-pressure wound therapy with instillation and dwell time: an overview. Plast Reconstr Surg 2021; 147(1S-1):16S–26S.
27. Weir D, Schultz G. Assessment and management of wound-related infections. In: Doughty DB, McNichol LL, editors. Wound, ostomy and continence nurses society core curriculum wound management. Philadelphia: Wolters Kluwer; 2016. p. 156–80.
28. Woo K, Dowsett C, Costa B, et al. Efficacy of topical cadexomer iodine treatment in chronic wounds: systematic review and meta-analysis of comparative clinical trials. Int Wound J 2021;18(5):586–97.
29. Amaya R. Use of polymeric membrane dressings for debridement of wounds in extreme premature infants <25 weeks gestation. Lecture presented at the 7th Annual Meeting of the International Society of Pediatric Wound Care. November 15, 2019; Houston, TX.

Comprehensive Management of Pressure Injury: A Review

Lyndsay A. Kandi, BS[a], India C. Rangel, BS[b],
Nellie V. Movtchan, MD[a], Nicole R. Van Spronsen, MD[a],
Erwin A. Kruger, MD[a],*

KEYWORDS

- Pressure injury • Pressure ulcer • Plastic surgery • Reconstruction
- NPIAP guidelines

KEY POINTS

- Pressure injuries (PIs) are multifactorial resulting in localized damage to the skin and underlying soft tissues, often requiring management by a multidisciplinary team.
- Nonsurgical management for PI stages 1 to 2 centers around pressure relief, wound debridement, control of local infection, and optimization of nutrition.
- PIs stages 3 to 4 typically require surgical debridement and possible reconstruction, with flap options generally based on anatomic location of the PI and ambulatory status.
- A major contributing factor to recurrence of PIs is inability to adequately off-load pressure consistently; thus, postoperative rehabilitation protocols are supplemented with support surfaces, specialty beds, and ultimately patient compliance with prevention strategies.
- Education of the patient on prevention is of utmost importance.

INTRODUCTION

Pressure injury (PI) wounds or PIs present a challenge to patients, caretakers, health care providers, and physicians due to their multifactorial etiologies and variable management. The ideal of multidisciplinary teams coordinating successful wound management is limited by factors within the inpatient health care system, the patient's socioeconomic status, and access to quality, patient-centric outpatient care. PIs arise most often from prolonged sustained pressure over a bony prominence resulting in ischemic tissue injury. Increased friction and shearing forces are exacerbated by patient's need to transfer with their underlying insensate, immobile, and possibly spastic

---

Financial Disclosure Statement: There are no financial conflicts of interest to disclose.
[a] Division of Plastic and Reconstructive Surgery, Department of Surgery, Mayo Clinic, Phoenix, AZ, USA; [b] Mayo Clinic Alix School of Medicine, Scottsdale, AZ, USA
* Corresponding author. Mayo Clinic, 5779 E. Mayo Boulevard, Phoenix, AZ 85054.
E-mail address: Kruger.Erwin@mayo.edu

Abbreviations	
CBC	Complete blood count
CMP	Comprehensive medical panel
CRP	C-reactive protein
HbA1C	Hemoglobin A1C
IV	Intravenous
CT	Computed tomography
HOB	Head of bed
SNF	Skilled nursing facility
LTAC	Long-term acute care
RN	Registered nurse

states. Patients with poor nutritional status, poor glycemic control, poor socioeconomic and family support, urinary and fecal incontinence, and location of the PI are just some of the factors that prolong wound healing and increase recurrence rates.[1,2] The incidence of PIs is highest among patients who are (1) elderly with neurologic impairment; (2) chronically hospitalized or in palliative care; and (3) under the age of 45 with spinal cord injuries.[1,3]

PIs range from a small area of non-blanchable erythema of intact skin to deep ulcerations extending to fascia, muscle, or bone. Despite adjusting for major comorbidities, PIs continue to be an independent predictor of mortality.[4] Not only are PIs devastating to the patient's quality of life, but they also contribute to enormous costs to the health care system (eg, recurrent hospitalizations, clinic visits, and resource utilization of outpatient nursing and home health care services). Current predictions of health care cost of PIs due to hospital-acquired PIs in the United States range from $17.8 billion to $26.8 billion.[5,6] Knowledge of factors contributing to the pathogenesis and development of PIs allows for early identification, prevention, and proper management of these complex wounds.

EPIDEMIOLOGY

A recent study conducted by Li and colleagues reported that the pooled prevalence of PIs among hospitalized adults was 12.8% globally. The incidence rate is 5.4 per 10,000 patient days,[7] whereas in the United States approximately 3 million adults experience PIs annually.[8] In a meta-analysis examining 5523 elderly patients, Song and colleagues found that patients with a PI had a twofold increased risk of mortality compared with controls.[9] In the United States, the estimated treatment cost has risen to $26.8 billion in the treatment of stage 3 or higher PIs, thus suggesting that early detection and subsequent action can result in large cost reduction.[5,6] In 2008, Medicare introduced a penalty for hospital-acquired PIs, adding them to a list of

Table 1
Summary of extrinsic factors that lead to the generation of a pressure injury[3,35]

Extrinsic Factor	Mechanism
Shear	Stretches muscle perforators to superficial tissues and may result in superficial necrosis
Pressure	Tissue deformation and resultant ischemia may result in deep necrosis
Friction	Loss of, or injury to, epidermis
Moisture	Skin maceration and breakdown

"preventable complications." However, despite the National Pressure Injury Advisory Panel (NPIAP) consensus that most PIs are preventable and Medicare attaching a financial consequence to hospital-acquired PIs, the incidence of hospital-acquired PIs has not changed.[10] As life expectancy and the world population ages,[11] the prevalence and incidence of the PIs may predictably increase as well.

PATIENT EVALUATION OVERVIEW
Assessment of Patient Comorbidities and Contributing Factors

Identification of underlying patient comorbidities is paramount to adequate treatment and prevention of PI occurrence and recurrence. Tissue injury is a result of both extrinsic and intrinsic factors, with the former related to mechanical forces on soft tissue and the latter based on the patient's physiologic factors and comorbidities (**Tables 1** and **2**). A risk assessment score with moderate predictive validity may consider is the Braden Scale, which considers a limited range of risk factors and sets a threshold for PI development in the context of different clinical environments.[12] The scale must be used in conjunction with clinical judgment.

An initial evaluation of the patient includes a comprehensive history and physical examination focused on PI history: onset, duration, progression, prior treatments, debridement, and reconstructions. An evaluation of the patient's functional capacity, ambulatory status, cognition, psychosocial support, and other social determinants of health such as health literacy and insurance coverage is all equally important considerations to develop a comprehensive wound management program. Laboratory and imaging studies may be ordered for completeness. A routine CBC, CMP, CRP, prealbumin, and HbA_1C are crucial for an initial evaluation of the patient's hematologic, infectious, nutritional, and glycemic baseline levels. Patients with PIs and chronic conditions may require further optimization of their underlying conditions and risk stratification by a subspecialist to maximize their potential to heal.

Pressure Injury Assessment and Staging Guidelines

The most widely accepted staging system for PIs was proposed by the NPIAP and has been revised several times since its introduction in 1989. The 2016 version identifies a PI as a "localized damage to the skin and underlying soft tissue usually over a bony prominence or related to a medical or other device" that may present as "intact skin

Table 2
Summary of intrinsic factors that lead to the generation of a pressure injury[3,35]

Intrinsic Factor	Mechanism
Ischemia (eg, vascular disease)	Decreased tissue perfusion may predispose to tissue necrosis
Decreased autonomic control	Spasms leading to prolonged contractures, excess perspiration, and lack of bladder or bowel control leading to increased moisture and skin breakdown
Increased age	Decreased tensile strength leading to increased friability
Decreased sensorineural, altered level of consciousness	Inability to appreciate discomfort from a prolonged position may result in tissue ischemia and necrosis
Anemia	May result in prolonged immobilization if anemia severe enough to cause weakness; decreased wound healing
Malnutrition	Decreased wound healing capabilities

Stages of Pressure Injuries

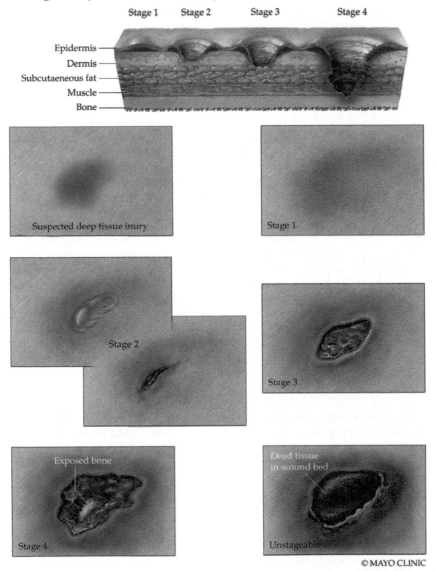

Stage 1   Stage 2   Stage 3   Stage 4

Epidermis
Dermis
Subcutaeneous fat
Muscle
Bone

Suspected deep tissue inury

Stage 1

Stage 2

Stage 3

Exposed bone

Dead tissue in wound bed

Stage 4

Unstageable

© MAYO CLINIC

Fig. 1. NPIAP guidelines for staging pressure injuries. (*From* Mayo Clinic Patient Education. Stages of Pressure Injuries (MC5896-02) Rochester, MN: Mayo Clinic, 2017, used with permission of Mayo Foundation for Medical Education and Research, all rights reserved.)

or an open ulcer."[13] Updated classifications provide a basic guideline for examination of wounds, including four distinct stages and two unstageable injuries (**Fig. 1**). After staging of a PI is determined via the NPIAP guidelines and therapy is initiated, proper documentation becomes an essential financial and legal component of the patient's medical record. A common practice is to refer to a PI as "healing stage X PI," otherwise confusion—and reimbursement issues—may ensue if a particular PI has several stages associated with it throughout the patient's medical record. Therefore, consistency in the documentation of the description of the wound, its dimensions, and progression is critical for proper management and reimbursement.

A useful supplementary tool is digital photography. Serial photographs help assess the changing dimensions and quality of the PI as well as unify the consensus among the various members of the interdisciplinary treatment team. Particularly in the setting of chronic wound management, patients require continuous monitoring of their clinical course; deviation from the projected course of healing, or contraction benchmark, may signal to the treating wound team or physician that treatment is inadequate and modifying the wound plan is warranted.

The updated NPIAP staging system concedes that the appearance of PIs may differ based on melanocytic integument—an issue that continues to lack guidance on the appropriate skin assessment protocols. Research on the intersection of PIs and healthcare disparities has concluded that despite significant literature on PIs, current staging guidelines do not effectively apply to darker skin tones. Superficial skin irritation and injury in patients with darker skin tones may not manifest as blanching erythema, but instead may present as hyperpigmentation or hypopigmentation. This issue has significant ramification for patients of darker skin tones who are more likely to develop higher stage PIs that are unrecognized.[14] To address this disparity in appearance of PIs on varying skin tones, various imaging techniques using alternate light source technologies have been proposed,[15–17] but are yet to become standard of care.

CONSERVATIVE TREATMENT OPTIONS

A basic knowledge of wound healing after tissue injury is needed to understand treatment options. The three phases—inflammation, proliferation, and maturation (**Fig. 2**)—each serve as a target of intervention. The inflammatory phase typically spans the first 6 days of healing and involves both vasoconstriction of damaged vessels and the recruitment of white blood cells to clear debris. Proliferation continues for the next few weeks and is characterized by reepithelialization and neovascularization of the injured tissue. The maturation phase begins around the third week of healing and is characterized by collagen deposition and remodeling leading to wound contraction and immature scar formation. Ultimately, the mature scar will have approximately 80% of the preinjury strength.[18] A chronic wound can stall at any phase of wound healing and serial debridement or advanced dressings aim to stimulate a wound environment back to a natural progression to the next phase. As a clinical benchmark, a wound should contract by area on average at a rate of 10% per week to a well-healed scar.

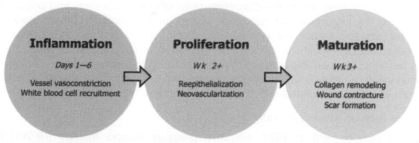

Fig. 2. The three stages of wound healing.

PIs occur secondary to the disruption of the physiologic processes of normal wound healing. Nonsurgical management for PI stages 1 to 2 centers around pressure relief, enzymatic wound debridement, control of local infection, and optimization of nutrition. Stages 3 to 4 typically require surgical debridement and possible reconstruction.[3]

Pressure Relief: Prevention and Treatment

Pressure relief can be achieved by specialized support surfaces, reducing pressure points, and implementing off-loading turning protocols for bedbound patients. For spinal cord injury patients, pressure relief protocols are based on the level of injury and amount of time in a wheelchair for self-guided home care prevention. Currently, NPIAP guidelines recommend individualized repositioning schedules for those who are at risk of developing PIs. These schedules take into account the individual's mobility and ability to reposition without assistance. However, these schedules place a large burden on the primary caretakers. This has led to an abundance of research investigating team-based methods for pressure relief, such as pre-intervention education, "turn teams,"[19] multidisciplinary teams,[20] and even wireless sensors for visual cueing of staff.[21]

Off-loading or turning protocols can be supplemented with advanced support surfaces and specialty beds.[22] The most recent advancements in specialized beds, specifically "robotic mattresses," have brought automatically regulated interface pressure mapping, aimed at improving both PI prevention and overall comfort,[23] but are not widespread in clinical practice to date.

Despite a large amount of research focused on determining which of the many pressure relief tools are most effective, there is no clear front-runner. In a large meta-analysis investigating support surfaces, McInnes and colleagues found that physically alternating patients to off-load pressure versus constant low-pressure devices did not significantly differ in terms of PI development. Furthermore, there was no significant difference between alternating pressure overlays versus mattresses, although mattresses were more likely to reduce costs.[22]

Local Wound Care

Local wound care is essential for proper healing of PIs. There are many options for local wound care, including topical antimicrobials, wound dressings, and solutions for cleansing or debriding the wound. With the rise of multidrug-resistant organisms colonizing wounds, topical or oral antibiotics should not be used preventatively. Antiseptic wound cleansing solutions, creams, or ointments, such as Dakin's solution (0.025% sodium hypochlorite), silver sulfadiazine, polyhexanide, and iodophors, are very effective and without conferring the risk of developing resistance.[24]

The choice of wound dressing is also a critical step in wound management and has high variability with limited high-quality research. The NPIAP guidelines largely leave choice in wound dressing to the discretion of health care providers and physicians, highlighting the importance of individual wound assessments.[25] General considerations for choosing a wound program assess biofilm, drainage, location of the wound, and periwound skin quality. Wound dressings are tailored to the wound needs, particularly the need for antimicrobial properties, absorption capacity, and the size, shape, and tunneling of the wound. Dressings should also consider the patient's access to supplies and cost associated with the wound program.

Negative Pressure Wound Therapy

Since its development in 1997, negative pressure wound therapy (NPWT) has emerged as a method of PI treatment. NPWT reduces the risk of infection and simplifies wound dressing changes,[26] both of which have been shown to positively affect the patient's quality of life.[27] The additional feature of topical fluid instillation and dwelling time has resulted in a lower number of surgical debridements and shorter hospital stays when compared with NPWT alone.[28] Despite the advancement and widespread use of NPWT, wound specialists should still use judgment and tailor the use of this technology based on the dynamic needs of the wound.

Debridement

Debridement of nonviable tissue is crucial for resetting a wound and setting the stage for progressive wound healing. Sharp debridement uses cutting devitalized tissue with scalpels, scissors, ring curettes, or advanced debridement technology/devices (eg, hydrosurgery jet). Mechanical or enzymatic debridement includes abrasion tools, curetting, wet-to-dry dressings, pulse lavage, biosurgical or maggot therapy, and enzymatic/chemical/collagenase ointments. Finally, surgical debridement uses a combination of the above in sedated or anesthetized patients and adds the advantage of obtaining deep tissue cultures or bone biopsies to guide antibiotic therapy.

Local Tissue Infection and Underlying Osteomyelitis

Open wounds, biofilm/slough, necrotic tissue, normal skin and enteric pathogen colonization, and exposure to multidrug-resistant organisms are all avenues that pressure wounds can develop local infection and underlying, chronic osteomyelitis.[29] Careful, repeated wound inspection, serial debridement, and tailored local wound care strategies are necessary to control bacterial colonization and/or infection. Globally, inappropriate use of wide-spectrum antibiotics has resulted in the emergence of antibiotic-resistant organisms in health care systems. Therefore, it is crucial to take measures to prevent wound infection, obtain meaningful cultures and deep bone biopsies of non-colonized bone, to then guide management, and prescribe targeted, evidence-based antibiotic courses.[30]

Treatment, incidence, and prevalence of clinically significant osteomyelitis in deep, chronic PI wounds remain controversial. The role of imaging in the diagnosis of osteomyelitis is similarly controversial in this setting, with studies showing that CT scans have a much lower sensitivity and specificity than bone biopsy.[31] MRI efficacy regarding osteomyelitis has the specificity of 22% despite a high sensitivity (94%). With bone biopsy remaining the gold standard for diagnosis of osteomyelitis, the role of preoperative MRI may assist with guiding the extent of surgical treatment.[32] IV antibiotics are crucial in the management of osteomyelitis, with most investigators recommending antibiotic therapy to 6 weeks or less.[32] Surgical debridement of stage 4 pressure ulcerations is an opportunity to obtain deep bone biopsies in a controlled environment to guide diagnosis and antibiotic treatment of osteomyelitis and should be recommended.

Nutrition

Nutrition is a key underlying factor contributing to wound healing, with nutritional status being a significant predictor of preventing or developing a PI.[25,33] In order to address this component of PIs, a comprehensive assessment by a nutritionist is recommended and has been shown to improve healing.[34] Intake of appropriate levels of protein, vitamins, and minerals should be optimized by a nutritionist and albumin and prealbumin levels should be monitored. For patients with PIs that are malnourished, the NPIAP strongly recommends implementing an individualized nutrition plan which includes 1.2 to 1.5 g protein/kg body weight/d. [25] Surgical candidacy for reconstruction of stage 4 PIs remains a clinical decision, but traditionally benchmarks of an

Table 3
Reconstruction options based on anatomic site of pressure injury[3,35,48]

PI Anatomic Site	Common Flaps	Blood Supply	Arc of Rotation	Special Considerations
Ischial	Gluteus *Musculocutaneous, muscle-only, fasciocutaneous (posterior/gluteal thigh flap)*	Inferior gluteal artery	Rotation, readvancement, island	Posterior/gluteal thigh flap may be used in ambulatory patients but gluteal flaps based on gluteus maximum muscle (fasciocutaneous) are inappropriate for ambulatory patients
	Hamstring (rectus femoris, semitendinosus, semimembranosus)	Profunda femoris perforators	V-Y advancement, readvancement	
	Gracilis *Fasciocutaneous, musculocutaneous*	Medial femoral circumflex artery		For a medially located defect
	TFL *Musculocutaneous, muscle-only*	Lateral femoral circumflex artery		
	Rectus abdominis			
Sacrum	Gluteus *fasciocutaneous, perforator, musculocutaneous*	Superior and/or inferior gluteal artery	V-Y advancement, rotation, island, readvancement	May be used in ambulatory patients
Trochanter	TFL *Perforator*	Lateral femoral circumflex artery	V-Y advancement, readvancement, transposition	
	Vastus lateralis	Descending branch of lateral circumflex femoral artery		
	Gluteus *Fasciocutaneous, myocutaneous, muscle-only*	Superior and/or inferior gluteal artery		For trochanteric PIs that communicate with hip joint
	Girdlestone procedure with vastus lateralis inclusion to fill dead space	Vastus lateralis: descending branch of lateral circumflex femoral artery		

Abbreviation: TFL, tensor fascia lata.

albumin greater than 3.0 g/dL and prealbumin greater than 15 mg/dL suggest a nutritional state amenable to surgical flap reconstruction.[1]

SURGICAL INTERVENTION

PI stages 3 and 4 commonly require operative management. An array of surgical modalities is available and largely depends on the anatomic location of the PI, prior surgery, and the patient's ambulatory status (**Table 3**).[35] Goals of reconstruction include complete debridement of devitalized tissue including bone, achievement of hemostasis, and obliteration of dead space. Flap selection should not jeopardize future flap options for coverage, and the suture line should be placed away from the area of direct pressure to prevent wound healing complications.

Although a surgical reconstruction may allow the patient to regain their activities of daily living thereby improving their quality of life, these reconstructions require commitment. All surgical patients face a physically and psychologically prolonged recovery, from an inpatient perioperative stay to an extended rehabilitation period, and then followed by indefinite outpatient surveillance. Patients also run the risk of recurrence. As with any procedure, informed consent of the risks and benefits and a discussion of expectations and recovery are required. Psychosocial support remains an important element when considering surgical procedures, particularly in the case of end-stage disease where patients may ultimately decide to undergo extremity amputation.

Postoperative management following flap-based reconstruction has been extensively reviewed in the literature and differs by institution. Generally, protocols aimed at optimizing patient comorbidities and risk factors are instituted preoperatively, targeting both intrinsic (eg, smoking cessation, nutritional supplementation, spasticity control, blood glucose control) and extrinsic (eg, relief of pressure, shear, friction, moisture control) factors. Duration of bed rest following surgery and sitting protocols vary in the literature and by institution, however follow general wound healing principles of adequate wound tensile strength achievement by postoperative week 6.[36] Although recent studies advocate for a more rapid sitting progression, bed rest for up to 6 weeks with complete pressure relief and repositioning in 2- to 4-hour intervals has historically been recommended.[37] With growing costs of health care utilization in the United States, a 6- to 8-week postoperative flap protocol needs to transition out of the inpatient facility appropriately and safely to long-term acute care facilities, short-term stay facilities, or in well-motivated and supported patients, tailored outpatient settings.

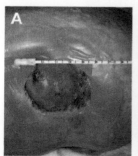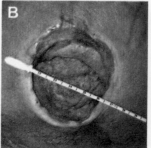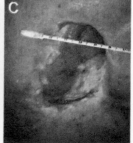

Fig. 3. (*A*) Preoperative left ischial PI before the Girdlestone procedure. (*B*) Preoperative right ischial PI following multiple debridements and NPWT therapy. (*C*) Preoperative sacral PI following multiple debridements and NPWT therapy.

CASE REPORT

A 54-year-old woman with a past medical history significant for complete T6 paraplegia spinal cord injury secondary to a skiing accident in 2000 presented for the evaluation of stage 4 sacral and bilateral ischial PIs after a decade of debridements and IV antibiotic treatments for underlying osteomyelitis. **Fig. 3** demonstrate the PIs immediately before definitive operative management. The patient used a specialty bed and negative pressure therapy throughout the years to aid in wound management. She followed a high-protein diet with vitamin supplementation.

She underwent CT imaging which demonstrated a direct communication between the left hip joint and septic trochanteric PI and was offered a left-sided Girdlestone procedure, antibiotic bead placement, and local tissue rearrangement for closure at the initial stage with a combined approach to her wound by orthopedic and plastic surgery. NPWT was reinstated to the bilateral ischial and sacral PIs after serial debridement. She was discharged to a care facility with drains with a plan for staged reconstruction after nutrition optimization. Once biopsy-proven osteomyelitis was diagnosed of her femur, infectious disease recommended 6 weeks of IV antibiotics.

She was readmitted to undergo removal of antibiotic beads, serial debridements of her stage 4 ischial, and sacral PIs with application of negative pressure therapy. The sacral defect measured 15 cm × 12 cm × 3 cm down to exposed sacral nerve roots; the right-sided ischial wound measured 7 cm × 7 cm and the left ischial wound was 10 cm × 8 cm. On staged admission, she was found to have failure to thrive in the outpatient setting without improvement in nutrition requiring supplemental tube feeds. She underwent multiple debridements with NPWT until nutritionally optimized to then stage her flap reconstructions as follows: a posterior thigh advancement flap, vastus lateralis advancement flap to the Girdlestone defect, right gluteal advancement flap, and left gluteal rotational flap (**Fig. 4**).

Difficulties in placement for her complex flap rehabilitation protocol prolonged an inpatient stay, with an eventual discharge to home with home health for flap recovery (low air loss mattress), nutritional optimization, daily skin checks and wound care, frequent 2 hour turns, and IV antibiotics. At her 2-month follow-up from discharge, she showed no signs of new PIs.

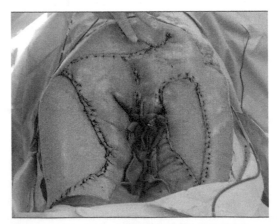

Fig. 4. Immediate postoperative photo following right gluteal advancement flap and left gluteal rotational flap.

Box 1
The postoperative flap protocol and rehabilitation guidelines used at our institution

Spinal cord injury pressure sore postoperative flap protocol and rehabilitation guidelines

The following is a summary of general guidelines for an 8-week pressure score flap reconstruction postoperative protocol:

Week 1: Bed rest on air-fluidized or fluid immersion bed. Patient supine with brief 30° HOB elevation for meals. Nutrition consult to co-follow as well as medical subspecialities as needed. Neurogenic bowel regimen and daily wound and drain care by plastic surgery team.

Week 2: Bed rest on air-fluidized or fluid immersion bed. Patient supine with brief 30° HOB elevation for meals. Nutrition optimization. Daily skin and wound care. Drains to be removed by surgical team when less than 30 cc/d × 48 hours. Transfer to SNF or LTAC with inpatient wound care team, flap protocol capabilities.

Week 3: Bed rest on air-fluidized or fluid immersion bed. Patient supine with brief 30° HOB elevation for meals. Nutrition optimization. Daily skin and wound care.

Week 4: Bed rest on air-fluidized or fluid immersion bed. Patient supine with brief 30° HOB elevation for meals. Nutrition optimization. Daily skin and wound care.

Week 5: Transfer to low air loss mattress with q2 hour turning by RN staff. Patient supine with brief 30° HOB elevation for meals. Nutrition optimization. Daily skin and wound care. Prone gurney upper body rehabilitation allowed under supervision for transfers in appropriate patient (eg, paraplegia with stable airway).

Week 6: Low air loss mattress with q2 hour turning by RN staff. Patient supine with brief 30° HOB elevation for meals. Nutrition optimization. Daily skin and wound care. Prone gurney upper body rehabilitation allowed under supervision for transfers in appropriate patient (eg, paraplegia with stable airway).

Week 7 to 8: Low air loss mattress with q2 hour turning by RN staff. Progressive sitting program under supervision by 15 minutes a day to a goal of 2 hours with q15 minute pressure reliefs under supervision. Complete rehabilitation, complete pressure mapping, and wheelchair/cushion evaluation and modifications as necessary. Comprehensive transition to home plan with outpatient home health, physical therapy, and follow-up plan.

Case Report Discussion and Flap Rehabilitation Protocol

The success of this complex surgical case is largely due to the main points reflected throughout this article: a multifactorial approach with a variety of interventions such as nutritional assessment and optimization; local wound care, including NPWT and repeated debridements; and operative management for late-stage PIs with the emphasis on pressure off-loading/use of specialty beds as well as the utilization of home health services. This approach is outlined throughout the 8-week postoperative flap protocol (**Box 1**) that the senior author (EAK) of this institution follows. The case also demonstrates that for complex cases, inpatient admission is often the only recourse to debride, prepare, and eventually close multiple PIs in debilitated patients.

NEW DEVELOPMENTS

To reduce the workload of health care workers while providing ever-improving care to patients, there has been a rise in the use of machine-learning technologies to prevent PIs. These methods include determining risk factors from electronic health records, posture recognition software, and machine learning analysis of PI images. These technologies are still in the early stages of development, with need for both external validation and research involving a wider range of PI patients; however, preliminary studies are promising.[38–41]

During the rise of the COVID-19 pandemic, less typical forms of PIs have become more prevalent, such as those due to face masks and prone positioning. This has called for pressure relief methods for N95s that may be implemented without disrupting the seal, the most successful of which were silicone dressings.[42] As for sedated and vented patients placed in the prone position, similar rules apply with regard to repositioning, dressing, and so forth as did with patients in the supine position. However, the large number of patients in this relatively uncommon position for long durations of time, along with complications such as intubations, poses a new challenge for health care providers.[43,44]

EVALUATION OF OUTCOMES AND COMPLICATIONS

Complication rates following reconstruction vary in the current literature, with rates differing based on treatment modality. The most commonly reported complications are wound healing issues such as dehiscence or recurrence, hematoma, seroma, and flap necrosis resulting in partial flap loss as well as infection.[12,45] A large systematic review within the last decade found no significant difference with regard to recurrence or complication rates between fasciocutaneous, musculocutaneous, and perforator flap-based reconstruction in the treatment of PIs.[45] For a patient with recurrent extensive ulceration despite a history of multiple previous failed flap reconstructions and Girdlestone procedures, their disease burden may be termed "end-stage." In this scenario, unilateral or bilateral disarticulation and total thigh or fillet flap reconstruction may be the patient's only option.

Recurrence continues to be the most important complication and is fairly common, although the true incidence is difficult to assess given lack of long-term outcome studies. Reports suggest that PU recurrence after flap reconstruction ranges from 15% to 82%,[1] and most commonly occurs within 1 year of treatment.[35] The most notable factor contributing to the recurrence of PIs is patient nonadherence to pressure relief protocols. Some studies report higher recurrence rates in patients who are unable to adequately off-load pressure, as is the case with paraplegic patients compared with non-paraplegics.[46] This may be due to differences in pressure distribution compared with ambulatory patients.[47] Further, stages 3 and 4 PIs are more likely to recur.[35] The same factors leading to the development of the initial PI may lead to subsequent PIs if they are not adequately addressed or if there are no pressure relief protocols in place. Thus, if recurrence does happen, the patient must be fully reevaluated to control any risk factors before proceeding with surgical intervention.

SUMMARY

PIs continue to present a challenge to patients, caretakers, health care providers, and physicians despite improvements in prevention and new technologies in wound care and surgical management. A multidisciplinary team composed of caretakers, nursing, health care providers, social works, and physicians is often necessary to successfully and comprehensively treat a PI. With the inclusion of PIs on the list of "never events" for hospitalized patients, policies aimed at education of patients and caregivers have been drafted with the key goal of preventative measures. Pressure off-loading, nutrition optimization, and patient surveillance may reduce the number of higher grade PIs. As the population ages, understanding the pathophysiology of PI development and comprehensive management in vulnerable patients will remain a topic of discussion.

CLINICS CARE POINTS

- Pressure injuries (PIs) are a multifactorial condition resulting in localized damage to the skin and underlying soft tissues, often necessitating management by a multidisciplinary team.

- Nonsurgical management for PI stages 1 to 2 centers around pressure relief, wound debridement, control of local infection, and optimization of nutrition.

- PIs stages 3 to 4 typically require surgical debridement and possible reconstruction, with flap options generally based on anatomic location of the PI and ambulatory status.

- The most notable factor contributing to recurrence of PIs is inability to adequately off-load pressure consistently.

- Education of the patient on prevention is of utmost importance.

REFERENCES

1. Keys KA, Daniali LN, Warner KJ, et al. Multivariate predictors of failure after flap coverage of pressure ulcers. Plast Reconstr Surg 2010;125(6):1725–34.
2. Thorne CH. Grabb and Smith's Plastic Surgery. 7th Edition. Philadelphia: Lippincott Williams & Wilkins; 2013.
3. Jannis JEO-RE. Essentials of plastic surgery. 2nd edition. New York: Thieme Medical Publishers; 2017.
4. Ferris A, Price A, Harding K. Pressure ulcers in patients receiving palliative care: A systematic review. Palliat Med 2019;33(7):770–82.
5. Hajhosseini B, Longaker MT, Gurtner GC. Pressure Injury. Ann Surg 2020;271(4): 671–9.
6. Padula WV, Delarmente BA. The national cost of hospital-acquired pressure injuries in the United States. Int Wound J 2019;16(3):634–40.
7. Li Z, Lin F, Thalib L, et al. Global prevalence and incidence of pressure injuries in hospitalised adult patients: A systematic review and meta-analysis. Int J Nurs Stud 2020;105:103546.
8. Mervis JS, Phillips TJ. Pressure ulcers: Pathophysiology, epidemiology, risk factors, and presentation. J Am Acad Dermatol 2019;81(4):881–90.
9. Song YP, Shen HW, Cai JY, et al. The relationship between pressure injury complication and mortality risk of older patients in follow-up: A systematic review and meta-analysis. Int Wound J 2019;16(6):1533–44.
10. Waters TM, Daniels MJ, Bazzoli GJ, et al. Effect of Medicare's nonpayment for Hospital-Acquired Conditions: lessons for future policy. JAMA Intern Med 2015; 175(3):347–54.
11. Woolf SH, Schoomaker H. Life Expectancy and Mortality Rates in the United States, 1959-2017. Jama 2019;322(20):1996–2016.
12. Ricci JA, Bayer LR, Orgill DP. Evidence-Based Medicine: The Evaluation and Treatment of Pressure Injuries. Plast Reconstr Surg 2017;139(1):275e–86e.
13. Edsberg LE, Black JM, Goldberg M, et al. Revised National Pressure Ulcer Advisory Panel Pressure Injury Staging System: Revised Pressure Injury Staging System. J Wound Ostomy Continence Nurs 2016;43(6):585–97.
14. Oozageer Gunowa N, Hutchinson M, Brooke J, et al. Pressure injuries in people with darker skin tones: A literature review. J Clin Nurs 2018;27(17–18):3266–75.
15. Aloweni FAB, Ang SY, Chang YY, et al. Evaluation of infrared technology to detect category I and suspected deep tissue injury in hospitalised patients. J Wound Care 2019;28(Sup12):S9–16.
16. Leachtenauer J, Kell S, Turner B, Newcomer C, Lyder C, Alwan M. A Non-Contact Imaging-Based Approach to Detecting Stage I Pressure Ulcers. Conference proceedings : Annual International Conference of the IEEE Engineering in Medicine

and Biology Society IEEE Engineering in Medicine and Biology Society Conference. 30 August – 03 September, 2006, New York.

17. Owens L, Warfield T, MacDonald R, et al. Using Alternative Light Source Technology to Enhance Visual Inspection of the Skin. J Wound Ostomy Continence Nurs 2018;45(4):356–8.

18. Wallace HA, Basehore BM, Zito PM. Wound Healing Phases. In: StatPearls. Treasure Island (FL): StatPearls Publishing.Copyright © 2021, StatPearls Publishing LLC.; 2021. Available at: https://www.ncbi.nlm.nih.gov/books/NBK470443/.

19. Harmon LC, Grobbel C, Palleschi M. Reducing Pressure Injury Incidence Using a Turn Team Assignment: Analysis of a Quality Improvement Project. J Wound Ostomy Continence Nurs 2016;43(5):477–82.

20. Miller MW, Emeny RT, Freed GL. Reduction of Hospital-acquired Pressure Injuries Using a Multidisciplinary Team Approach: A Descriptive Study. Wounds 2019; 31(4):108–13.

21. Yap TL, Kennerly SM, Horn SD, et al. TEAM-UP for quality: a cluster randomized controlled trial protocol focused on preventing pressure ulcers through repositioning frequency and precipitating factors. BMC Geriatr 2018;18(1):54.

22. McInnes E, Jammali-Blasi A, Bell-Syer SE, et al. Support surfaces for pressure ulcer prevention. Cochrane Database Syst Rev 2015;2015(9):Cd001735.

23. Saegusa M, Noguchi H, Nakagami G, et al. Evaluation of comfort associated with the use of a robotic mattress with an interface pressure mapping system and automatic inner air-cell pressure adjustment function in healthy volunteers. J Tissue Viability 2018;27(3):146–52.

24. Kramer A, Dissemond J, Kim S, et al. Consensus on Wound Antisepsis: Update 2018. Skin Pharmacol Physiol 2018;31(1):28–58.

25. Prevention and Treatment of Pressure Ulcers/Injuries: Quick Reference Guide. In: European Pressure Ulcer Advisory Panel NPIAPaPPPIA, ed2019.

26. Han G, Ceilley R. Chronic Wound Healing: A Review of Current Management and Treatments. Adv Ther 2017;34(3):599–610.

27. Janssen AH, Wegdam JA, de Vries Reilingh TS, et al. Negative pressure wound therapy for patients with hard-to-heal wounds: a systematic review. J Wound Care 2020;29(4):206–12.

28. Arowojolu OA, Wirth GA. Sacral and Ischial Pressure Ulcer Management With Negative-Pressure Wound Therapy With Instillation and Dwell. Plast Reconstr Surg 2021;147(1s-1):61s–7s.

29. Braga IA, Pirett CC, Ribas RM, et al. Bacterial colonization of pressure ulcers: assessment of risk for bloodstream infection and impact on patient outcomes. J Hosp Infect 2013;83(4):314–20.

30. Karam G, Chastre J, Wilcox MH, et al. Antibiotic strategies in the era of multidrug resistance. Crit Care 2016;20(1):136.

31. Larson DL, Gilstrap J, Simonelic K, et al. Is there a simple, definitive, and cost-effective way to diagnose osteomyelitis in the pressure ulcer patient? Plast Reconstr Surg 2011;127(2):670–6.

32. Wong D, Holtom P, Spellberg B. Osteomyelitis Complicating Sacral Pressure Ulcers: Whether or Not to Treat With Antibiotic Therapy. Clin Infect Dis 2018;68(2): 338–42.

33. Yap J, Holloway S. Evidence-based review of the effects of nutritional supplementation for pressure ulcer prevention. Int Wound J 2021;18(6):805–21.

34. Allen B. Effects of a comprehensive nutritional program on pressure ulcer healing, length of hospital stay, and charges to patients. Clin Nurs Res 2013;22(2): 186–205.

35. O A. Michigan Manual of Plastic Surgery. 2 ed2014.
36. Ireton JE, Unger JG, Rohrich RJ. The role of wound healing and its everyday application in plastic surgery: a practical perspective and systematic review. Plast Reconstr Surg Glob Open 2013;1(1):e10–9.
37. Bergstrom N, Horn SD, Rapp MP, et al. Turning for Ulcer ReductioN: a multisite randomized clinical trial in nursing homes. J Am Geriatr Soc 2013;61(10): 1705–13.
38. Jiang M, Ma Y, Guo S, et al. Using Machine Learning Technologies in Pressure Injury Management: Systematic Review. JMIR Med Inform 2021;9(3):e25704.
39. Nakagami G, Yokota S, Kitamura A, et al. Supervised machine learning-based prediction for in-hospital pressure injury development using electronic health records: A retrospective observational cohort study in a university hospital in Japan. Int J Nurs Stud 2021;119:103932.
40. Ting JJ, Garnett A. E-Health Decision Support Technologies in the Prevention and Management of Pressure Ulcers: A Systematic Review. Comput Inform Nurs 2021;39(12):955–73.
41. Bogie KM, Roggenkamp SK, Zeng N, et al. Development of Predictive Informatics Tool Using Electronic Health Records to Inform Personalized Evidence-Based Pressure Injury Management for Veterans with Spinal Cord Injury. Mil Med 2021;186(Suppl 1):651–8.
42. Smart H, Opinion FB, Darwich I, et al. Preventing Facial Pressure Injury for Health Care Providers Adhering to COVID-19 Personal Protective Equipment Requirements. Adv Skin Wound Care 2020;33(8):418–27.
43. Moore Z, Patton D, Avsar P, et al. Prevention of pressure ulcers among individuals cared for in the prone position: lessons for the COVID-19 emergency. J Wound Care 2020;29(6):312–20.
44. Peko L, Barakat-Johnson M, Gefen A. Protecting prone positioned patients from facial pressure ulcers using prophylactic dressings: A timely biomechanical analysis in the context of the COVID-19 pandemic. Int Wound J 2020;17(6):1595–606.
45. Sameem M, Au M, Wood T, et al. A systematic review of complication and recurrence rates of musculocutaneous, fasciocutaneous, and perforator-based flaps for treatment of pressure sores. Plast Reconstr Surg 2012;130(1):67e–77e.
46. Evans GR, Dufresne CR, Manson PN. Surgical correction of pressure ulcers in an urban center: is it efficacious? Adv Wound Care 1994;7(1):40–6.
47. Brienza DM, Karg PE. Seat cushion optimization: a comparison of interface pressure and tissue stiffness characteristics for spinal cord injured and elderly patients. Arch Phys Med Rehabil 1998;79(4):388–94.
48. Cushing CA, Phillips LG. Evidence-based medicine: pressure sores. Plast Reconstr Surg 2013;132(6):1720–32.

Seating and Wheeled Mobility Clinicians Contribute to the Wound Care Team

Cathy H. Carver, MS, PT, ATP/SMS[a],*, Stacey Mullis, OTR/L, ATP[b],
Kathleen H. Fitzgerald, PT, DPT, NCS[c]

KEYWORDS

- Pressure injury • Wheelchair user • Seating and wheeled mobility clinic
- Seating system • Pressure mapping • Complex rehabilitation technology

KEY POINTS

- An OT/PT as the seating and wheeled mobility (SWM) specialist has expertise beyond prevention of pressure injuries and should be included in the wound care team to provide additional interventions to manage existing pressure injuries.
- Addressing wounds of a wheelchair user requires more than just consideration of the cushion and pressure mapping. The seating system as a whole can affect the onset and healing of pressure injuries.
- The SWM evaluation is an extensive examination of the wheelchair user's current equipment, intrinsic and extrinsic factors, and function. A comprehensive assessment is required to make appropriate recommendations for equipment modification or replacement.

INTRODUCTION

People with various disabilities need to monitor their skin to maintain their health Appendix 1 Those who become unable to walk and use a wheelchair (WC) are at higher risk for injury to their skin. Wheelchair users are susceptible to pressure, shear, moisture, or other potential causes of skin injury. Avoiding being in the WC is not an option as sitting is key to nutritional intake, toileting, communication, mobility, socialization, and overall psychological health. Access to clinicians who can help with wound healing is paramount. The wound care team involves physicians and nurses

[a] UAB/Spain Rehabilitation Center, 1717 6th Avenue South R151, Birmingham, AL 35249, USA;
[b] Anthros, 416 Bluemound Road, Waukesha, WI, 53188, USA; [c] Department of Physical Therapy, Faulkner University, 5345 Atlanta Hathway, Montgomery, AL 36109, USA
* Corresponding author.
E-mail address: ccarver@uabmc.edu

Phys Med Rehabil Clin N Am 33 (2022) 789–803
https://doi.org/10.1016/j.pmr.2022.06.011
1047-9651/22/© 2022 Elsevier Inc. All rights reserved.

who specialize in surgical procedures, topical care, wound dressings, and pharmaceuticals to improve wound healing. The National Pressure Injury Advisory Panel (NPIAP) Clinical Practice Guideline (CPG) for wound care[1] addresses the various aspects of wound healing and states that immobility is a major risk factor for pressure injury. Individuals who have difficulty with mobility may use a WC, which increases their risk of pressure injury. One way of assisting at-risk WC users is having their wheelchair and seating system assessed by an occupational therapist (OT) or a physical therapist (PT), who is familiar with the principles of seating and wheeled mobility (SWM). Many of these skilled OTs and PTs are credentialed by the Rehabilitation Engineering and Assistive Technology Society of North America (RESNA) as an Assistive Technology Professional (ATP) or additionally as a Seating and Mobility Specialist (SMS).

The ability of people who are nonambulatory to obtain WCs, specifically complex rehabilitation technology (CRT), which is individually configured mobility equipment, has improved over the last several years due to improved accessibility, inclusion efforts, and technology. Until the development of CRT, basic durable medical equipment (DME) types of WCs were the most common options (**Table 1**). The clinical skills of PTs and OTs to address specific needs of these individuals have also developed along with the technology of related products. Today, topics covered in some academic programs provide the foundation for participation in wound care management, specifically from the WC and seating perspective.[2] With the development of education and credentialing in SWM services, more expertise is available to thoroughly address someone with a disability using a WC long term.[3] This article will focus on this area of practice for the PT and OT as an SWM clinician, the assessment process for those with current skin injury, and how SWM clinicians work together with the wound care team.

LITERATURE REVIEW

Mounting literature is available citing the role of a PT or OT in performing wound care interventions or separately providing their expertise on mobility and posture as a part of the multidisciplinary team approach to pressure injuries.[5] Even more evidence can be found on the effectiveness of various support surfaces as they relate to pressure injuries.[6] However, there are fewer peer reviewed publications that document the role of the seating and mobility specialist as a part of the interdisciplinary wound care team.[7] A clinician who performs a comprehensive examination of current equipment and the specific extrinsic factors of the individual with a skin injury is critical to the resolution of pressure injuries and their recurrence.

COMMON MISCONCEPTIONS ABOUT WHEELCHAIRS AND PRESSURE INJURIES

The most common assumption regarding the onset of a pressure injury in a full-time WC user is that they are using the wrong WC cushion. However, all extrinsic and intrinsic factors related to the user must be considered when evaluating the seating system (**Table 2**). Too commonly pressure mapping alone without a comprehensive evaluation falls short in providing an appropriate evidence-based intervention. This article offers a more holistic approach that protects individuals at risk for skin injury.

IMPACT OF THE WHEELCHAIR SEATING SYSTEM ON SKIN INJURY

To demonstrate why the SWM therapist is a critical part of the interdisciplinary wound team for the WC user, one should consider how the seating system impacts skin injury

Table 1
DME and CRT defined according to Centers for Medicare and Medicaid[4]

Type of Equipment	Criteria	What Is Required by Medicare?
Durable medical equipment (DME)	Able to withstand repeated use Used for a medical purpose Not usually useful to someone who is not sick, injured, or disabled Used in the home	Prescription from physician and recent examination documenting the need for a mobility device No PT/OT evaluation or ATP involvement required Specific justification of the product may come from the physician or therapist On-site home evaluation not required
Complex rehabilitation technology (CRT)	Medically necessary, individually configured Manual Wheelchairs (MWCs), Power Wheelchairs (PWCs), adaptive seating systems, and other related technology Require evaluation, fitting, configuration, adjustment, or programming Designed to meet specific and unique medical, physical, and functional needs of individuals with a primary diagnosis resulting from a congenital disorder, progressive or degenerative neuromuscular disease, or injury/trauma	A broader range of services compared to DME Physician order and recent examination documenting the need for a mobility device Requires credentialed professionals such as an ATP Requires PT/OT evaluation, measurements, trials, fittings, training and education, and ongoing modifications Specific justification of the product may come from the physician or therapist CRT companies must comply with rigorous quality standards under Medicare

Abbreviations: ATP, assistive technology professional; OT, occupational therapist; PT, physical therapist; PWC, power wheelchair.

and healing. It is also important to understand the role of pressure and shear that contributes to cell deformation and death. **Fig. 1** shows the potential areas of pressure and shear in the seated posture.

Pressure: Pressure is a continuous force applied on or against an object by something in contact with it. This can create high peak pressures over bony prominences increasing the risk of skin breakdown. Traditionally, the extrinsic factor of pressure has been a primary focus to address to improve wound healing. Studies have shown that prolonged pressure leads to decreased oxygenation to the cells and eventually ischemia and cell death.[8] This happens over a period of hours and in most cases can be improved by repositioning and relieving the pressure in that area.

Shear: Shear is most simply understood as the combination of downward pressure and static friction.[9] What makes shear an insidious extrinsic factor is that it can happen unintentionally during weight shifts, reaching, or repositioning. It happens at the

Table 2	
Intrinsic and extrinsic factors that impact skin integrity	
Intrinsic factors	Age-related skin changes; poor nutrition and hydration; urinary and fecal incontinence; limited mobility; impaired sensation; postural deformities; impaired circulation; obesity/underweight; limited alertness; muscle spasms; smoking
Extrinsic factors	prolonged pressure, shear, and impaired microclimate

deeper levels of tissues, which means when it is noticed at the skin surface, the damage is irreversible. The skin around the pelvis could be analogous to a gelatinous sack. When an individual reaches for something and the outer skin "sticks" to the surface while the bony prominences underneath move, this causes stress and strain to the tissue and cells around it (**Fig. 2**). This stress and strain lead to cell deformation. Cell deformation needs to be better understood as it is more detrimental and causes irreversible damage at the cellular level and acts much faster than ischemia alone.

Three mechanisms that can result in cell death:

1. Distortion of the cell membrane: The membrane that separates the interior of the cells from the outside environment is damaged. The cell membrane's simple function is to protect the cell from its surroundings and regulate what comes in and goes out.
2. Disruption of cytoskeleton: The breakdown of the network of proteins (microfilaments and microtubules), which provides the internal shape and structural support to a cell.[10]
3. Decrease in pH: Once the cell membrane and cytoskeleton have been compromised, cellular pH can decrease. If wound healing is to be initiated or assisted, it is important that the wound bed pH be maintained above 4. However, when the

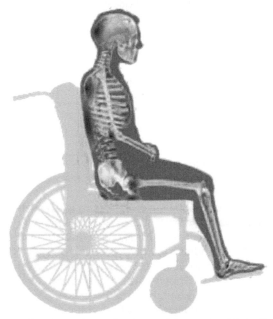

Fig. 1. High-risk areas for skin injury when seated in a wheelchair (in *red*). (*Courtesy of Permobil.*)

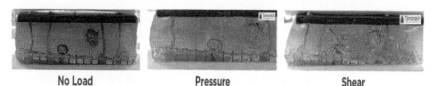

| No Load | Pressure | Shear |

Fig. 2. Cellular view of the application of pressure and friction. (*Courtesy of* Permobil.)

cell is damaged, the pH may drop into highly acidic levels, preventing wound healing.[11,12]

Microclimate: Microclimate is the state of moisture and temperature at the seat surface that contacts the individual. High moisture and high temperatures can contribute to the development or affect the healing of pressure injuries. Microclimate can be influenced by various factors, such as the material of the cushion and cover, outside temperature, infrequent repositioning, and incontinence to name a few.

DETERMINING THE BEST APPROACH TO SKIN HEALTH IN THE SEATED POSITION

Wound care clinicians are experts at understanding methods of pressure redistribution, namely, immersion and offloading of support surfaces, such as mattresses (**Table 3**). SWM therapists understand these principles in relation to various postures in a sitting position and evaluate in light of the entire seating system. Positioning and material selection by the SWM use the principles of offloading and immersion to optimize pressure distribution while maximizing functional mobility and independence of the WC user. These clinical decisions are dependent upon a comprehensive examination of the WC user.

PRESSURE MAPPING

One tool used to assess the WC and seating configuration is a pressure mapping system (Appendix 1). These systems can be a key tool to provide a snapshot in time of high peak pressures caused by postures and equipment or to identify high-risk areas. A pressure map uses advanced sensor technology to measure and visualize the pressure between the individual and the surface. The pressure is measured in millimeters of mercury (mm Hg) and presented as a colored image on a screen (**Fig. 3**). It should be noted that there is no threshold pressure that indicates risk according to the International Organization for Standardization (ISO).[13] This means that pressure mapping is useful to compare different products or configurations to determine which offers the least high peak pressures and best pressure distribution. These images provide a snapshot in time of how WC equipment choices and the configuration are increasing

Table 3	
Methods of pressure redistribution: offloading and immersion	
Offloading	The principle of redirecting pressure from a small surface area to a greater surface area that can withstand more pressure to prevent unwanted skin breakdown.[1]
Immersion	The principle of conforming to the person's shape by "sinking into" the medium. This promotes pressure redistribution over a larger surface area, minimizing high peak pressures at the bony prominences.[1]

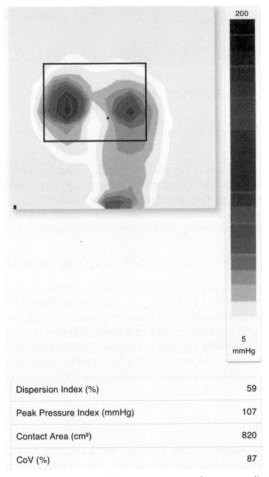

Dispersion Index (%)	59
Peak Pressure Index (mmHg)	107
Contact Area (cm²)	820
CoV (%)	87

Fig. 3. Pressure mapping equipment and image capture of pressure distribution.

or decreasing pressure over the bony prominences.[14] It does not calculate or measure other factors impacting skin injury, like shear, moisture, or other factors discussed above. It is only applied to the surfaces used in that moment. To obtain accurate readings, an individual must be pressure mapped in the seating system they use regularly or in the system they are concerned that could be causing skin injuries.

WHEN SHOULD PRESSURE MAPPING BE USED?

1. Persistent pressure injury: A pressure map can be used to help determine the source of the problem. The therapist can check pressure areas with adjustments to the configuration such as back angles or lower extremity positioning to determine the best configuration to manage pressure distribution.
2. Biofeedback: A pressure map is an excellent tool to show wheelchair users how effective their pressure relieving techniques are in allowing blood flow to problem areas. An individual can be taught effective pressure relieving strategies dependent upon the type of wheelchair they use such as leaning forward or leaning to one side or using power tilt in a power wheelchair to offload the bony areas of the pelvis. The

individual can be watching the screen and see how far they need to lean or tilt to achieve an effective pressure relief.

3. Secondary medical issues: Clinicians must consider diagnoses and the impact of aging skin, which may result in decreased tissue integrity. Some secondary medical issues, such as diabetes, are known to slow down the healing process. Metabolic imbalances and certain medications can also delay the healing process. In these cases, it is best to pressure-map the individual and determine if there are higher peak pressure areas that are at risk for breakdown and consider the impact of these comorbidities on healing.

4. Poor sensation: When someone has little or no sensation, they are at risk for skin injury as they do not have the sensory cue of pain or discomfort to provide warning of cell injury. In this case, a pressure map can help identify an appropriate cushion and identify potential areas of breakdown. Training in effective pressure relieving techniques as mentioned above is important. For the WC user who has normal or heightened sensation, comfort and function of the person should be strongly considered along with the pressure mapping to maximize compliance. For example, if an individual pressure-maps well on a cushion but is uncomfortable or they cannot balance while on it, they will inevitably abandon the cushion.

ROADMAP TO THE SEATING AND WHEELED MOBILITY CLINIC AND SERVICES OFFERED

For some with a chronic disability, noticing a skin injury that is healing slower than expected may prompt that person to seek medical attention. However, for many others the path to medical care is indirect. The person who identifies a skin injury or pending problem can vary as much as the cause of the wound itself. A caregiver may notice it while assisting with bathing; a wheelchair supplier making a delivery may notice drainage or odor from an area of concern; or an individual who attends the wheelchair clinic for an assessment may mention the onset of a pressure injury over a bony area that he/she has been treating at home off and on for over a year yet has never discussed with his physician. At any of these points, a referral can be made to a wound clinic for full medical evaluation and a subsequent plan of care for healing. If the individual is a full-time WC user, a referral to an SWM clinician skilled in CRT and seating assessments is recommended (**Fig. 4**).

THE COMPREHENSIVE SEATING AND WHEELED MOBILITY EVALUATION FOR THE WHEELCHAIR USER

Each topic addressed in the evaluation can be expanded upon according to individual findings/priorities/needs. A case example will follow to show how the below topics are addressed.

1. Chart review: Review medical records for history, prior/current treatment and plan of care, and any intrinsic factors (see **Table 2**).

2. Subjective interview: Upon initiating the appointment and a review of medical records that may or may not be available, a patient interview is conducted with the wheelchair user as well as any caregivers who may also be involved. While collecting subjective information, the SWM therapist observes movements or lack thereof while in the WC. Movements that occur due to sliding, spasms, pain, or dystonia are noted along with any self-initiated attempts to relieve pressure from sitting. If this has not occurred after 20 minutes of the initial exam, the SWM therapist can reason that the consumer likely does not move much at home. These observations

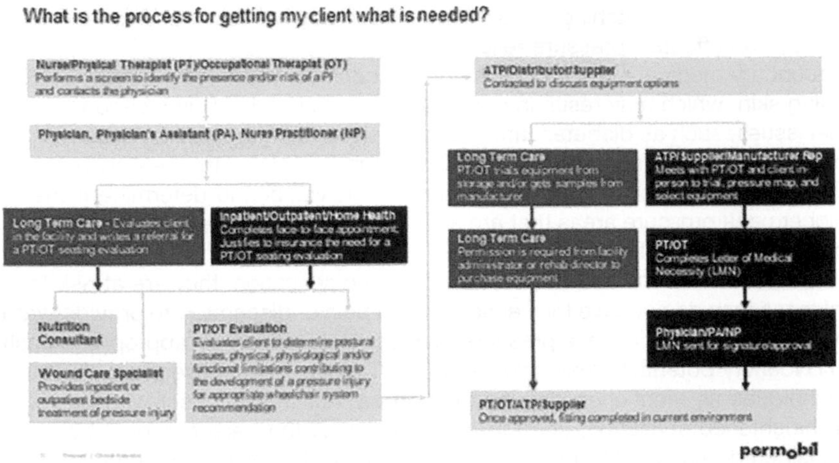

Fig. 4. The process of getting CRT equipment in different settings (Free download available of "The Wheelchair Seating Pocket Guide" for more information on the process of getting equipment: https://hub.permobil.com/permobil-resources). (*Courtesy of* Permobil.)

can provide valuable information to supplement the information collected during the examination. Subjective questions such as the following may be asked:

- Time since onset of wound(s)?
- Location and stage of wound(s)?
- Perceived caused your wound(s)?
- History of prior wound(s) and/or treatment by an MD, Doctor of Osteopathic medicine (DO) or Certified Registered Nurse Practitioner (CRNP)?
- Surgical interventions?
- Prior successful efforts to promote healing?
- Specific causes of exacerbations?
- Weight loss/gain?
- Changes in overall health or new medical conditions (including secondary medical conditions)?
- How do you transfer in/out of your WC ensuring no trauma to bony areas during transfers?[15]

3. 24-hour assessment/subjective information: It is important to discuss any and all positions or surfaces a person spends their time that may have contributed to the skin injury such as alternative WCs, cushions, or other sitting surfaces within the home or community settings. Seating surfaces in vehicles and work and school environments should also be considered. It is also important to consider sleeping surfaces and other DME such as shower seats/bench, transfer devices, and toileting aids for self-care tasks. One recommendation can be to have the consumer list (or bring photos) of all the places they sit or lie on and the type of surfaces and their condition. The use of these should be discussed to determine the length of time someone is in those positions and any potential for cause of pressure injury/shearing/excessive moisture. Caregivers can provide insight into daily function and observations such as transfer methods and activities that could be contributing to the pressure injury onset and healing status.

Example questions/Topics to discuss:

1. Sleep position and surface
2. Other places you sit–other WCs or surfaces, vehicle seats etc.

   3. Other DME used–toilet seat or shower chair (hard plastic?)
   4. Other environments–work, school, other homes...
   5. Other caregiver's input/assistance
   6. Type of clothing/undergarments used

4. Current WC and seating system: The fit, configuration and condition of the current WC seating system affects how pressure is distributed across the body (**Figs. 5** and **6**). **Table 4** provides examples of the components that will be assessed by the therapist to address possible causes of pressure and shear that can result in skin injury. As we consider equipment choices, the therapist is considering the intrinsic factors and extrinsic factors of pressure injury development. The medical records may inform the therapist of the intrinsic factors, but the extrinsic factors (see **Table 2**) will be assessed during the clinic visit. The fit may be affected by tissue length, flexibility, joint range of motion, spasticity, and spinal posture, which are also included in the objective assessment performed via a mat assessment by the therapist. Standard tools of assessment such as calipers and goniometer assist to evaluate for optimal configuration to promote function, stability, and pressure redistribution of the seating system.[16,17] The age of the system, any need for repairs and eligibility for changes through the consumer's funding source should be assessed. The CRT supplier will be able to assist with this information:

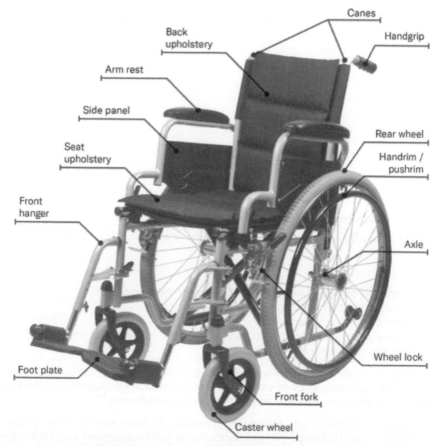

Fig. 5. Components of a manual wheelchair. (*Courtesy of* Permobil.)

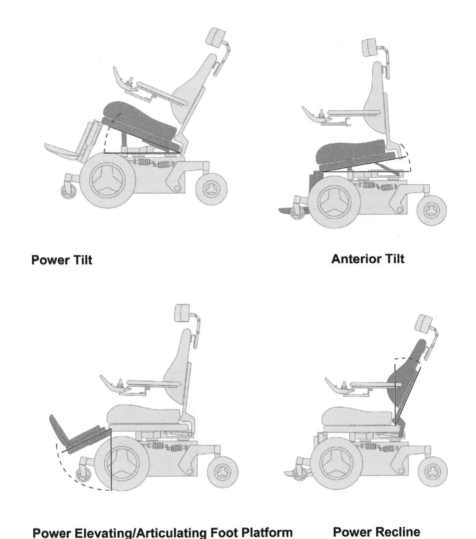

Power Tilt   **Anterior Tilt**

Power Elevating/Articulating Foot Platform   **Power Recline**

Fig. 6. Power functions for repositioning in a power wheelchair. (*Courtesy of* Permobil.)

- Information on age fit and appropriateness of the primary WC
- Address any other WCs used
- Age and wear of current seating
- Address any modifications or repairs needed with supplier and eligibility for funding of any recommendations

For those in power wheelchairs (PWCs), it is also required to assess the current functional use and frequency of use of the power functions if available on the PWC as these may affect the position and fit of seating components.[18]

5. Objective mat evaluation: Hands-on evaluation of bony prominences, postural tendencies, and tolerated external supports cannot be assessed when in the current system. Therefore, to evaluate a person's posture and support system needs,

Table 4
Common causes of abnormal sitting related to a person's fit in a WC

Manual Wheelchair	What to Look for
Seat width	Too wide: leaning to one side can result in pressure in unintended areas Too narrow: can result in pressure where buttocks/thighs overhang the cushion
Seat depth	Too short: poor pressure distribution through the thighs Too deep: Increased pressure from a posterior pelvic tilt and kyphotic posture
Seat slope	Too little: sliding, sacral sitting Too much: excessive pressure on ITs
Height of the footplates	Too high: thighs raised off the cushion and creating high peak pressures on the ITs Too low: creates pressure at the posterior distal thigh
Armrest height	Too high: poor neck/shoulder posture and pain, pressure on the elbows Too low: posterior postural tendencies and pressure in unintended areas

Abbreviation: ITs: ischial tuberosities.

an examination of posture, range of motion, pelvic and spinal alignment, and mobility must be completed with the person out of the chair on a mat table.[19]
6. Address extrinsic factors
   1. Microclimate
   2. Shear
   3. Prolonged pressure
7. Pressure mapping
8. Equipment trial
9. Education and recommendations: One of the most valuable interventions a skilled PT and OT can provide is patient and caregiver education. SWM therapists have the opportunity to reinforce all health factors the rest of the team is encouraging as well. Skin care is a life-long component of wellness and health maintenance, especially for individuals who are full-time WC users. This non-negotiable portion of their self-care demands increased diligence after the onset of a pressure injury. The seating clinician is frequently educating on topics such as the correct use of support surfaces, skin checks and signs of potential issues, and the method and frequency of effective pressure relief practices specific to this individual. Although these areas of education are anticipated, the comprehensive clinical exam can identify other possible factors that contribute to skin health. These may include care and cleaning of support surfaces, transfer technique and equipment used for transfers, edema management, scar tissue care and anatomical changes after surgical interventions, toileting programs, clothing choices that can contribute to shear or effect the microclimate, the use of other nonmedical support surfaces such as exercise equipment or transportation vehicles, and the effects of aging on posture and skin.[20] Each of these variables can contribute to healing and recurrence rates of pressure and shear injuries. During the exam a therapist is able to provide WC users and their caregivers with education, they can also identify areas that require referral to additional medical team members for further resources or interventions.
10. Documentation and communication with the team on findings: Documentation from the WC and seating clinic should include the reason for the visit, current

functional level, and a summary of topics discussed to determine any impact on the wound healing process. A summary of the current WC and seating system and any adjustments or changes needed should be justified. If pressure mapping was done, those findings should be objectively noted and any changes made after that along with education provided.

CASE EXAMPLE

A 21-year-old man was injured in a motorcycle accident that resulted in a C7 SCI. He weighed 225 pounds and was 6'1" tall at the time of his accident and was active and worked part-time in construction and was taking college classes. He was in the hospital for 4 weeks then inpatient rehabilitation for 3 more weeks. He had state Medicaid insurance at the time of his accident and went home from inpatient rehabilitation in a recliner manual wheelchair with a 2" foam cushion, sling back and elevating leg rests. He lived in a small town. His rental WC turned into a purchased item after 12 months. Eighteen months after his injury, he returned to see his rehabilitation MD and now weighs 170 pounds, has developed a stage 3 pressure injury on his sacrum and has contractures in his shoulders and ankles. He gets referred to the seating and wheeled mobility clinic for a WC and seating evaluation.

Review Medical Record for History, Treatment and Plan of Care and Any Intrinsic Factors

The patient has a stage 3 pressure injury on his sacrum and he is following up in the wound clinic monthly for dressing changes, and muscle flap surgery is being considered. The nutritional assessment shows low protein and the team recommends increased intake through diet and supplements. He smokes half a pack of cigarettes per day.

Subjective Questions

The patient reports the skin injury started 6 months ago on his "tailbone" and he has not had pressure injuries before. He is seeing the team in the wound clinic monthly. He thinks the wound was caused by being in bed a lot, depression, weight loss, and not a good seating system/WC. He also reports his bladder and bowel management is not consistent. He confirmed he does smoke half a pack per day to manage stress. He requires maximum assistance for his activities of daily living and transfers by mechanical lift. Observations while gathering information: Flexor and extensor spasms are noted and his clothing includes a large t-shirt and large blue jeans twisted around his hips because they are too big. He does not attempt or request assistance for pressure relief.

24-Hour Assessment/Subjective Information to Gather

He sleeps on his side in a semielectric hospital bed with a low–air-loss mattress. The only other place he sits is in a car seat to MD appointments. He does not use other DME at this time because he is bathed in bed, and his bowel and bladder program are done in bed. He is mainly at home now but hopes to continue to college classes and work again. His caregivers are his mother, grandmother, and a caregiver from the state waiver program and they report, "I can't get him to eat much; these spasms are hard to manage." He uses adult diapers and wears large blue jeans, athletic shorts, and t-shirts for his typical clothing.

Address Current Wheelchair and Seating System for Fit, Wear, Damage, Etc.

He is currently in a manual recliner wheelchair 18″ × 16″ in size with removable armrests, elevating leg rests, 2″ foam cushion, and vinyl backrest with a vinyl headrest. He does not have/use any other wheelchairs at this time. This wheelchair is 18 months old, and he is unable to push it; it does not support his posture; the seat depth is too short, and the elevating leg rests are not properly adjusted or used. His knees are higher than his hips and promote him sitting posteriorly ("sacral sitting"). His wheelchair is under 5 years old but he is functionally unable to use it and the seating is not meeting his postural needs or needs for pressure relief and positioning. Due to the change in condition of weight loss, onset of stage 3 sacral pressure injury and contractures, the SWM team will pursue a new WC and seating system.

Address Extrinsic Factors

Regarding microclimate, moisture is a factor from the use of adult diapers and sweating from autonomic dysreflexia. Shear is an issue from his spasticity. Of note he is unable to do an independent pressure relief due to weakness, shoulder contractures, and poor posture and absent trunk control.

Pressure Mapping

He will be pressure-mapped in the recommended PWC with power functions on a variety of cushions for his education and to ensure he is gets good distribution of pressure and determine if off-loading or immersion is the best approach for his pressure relief. The readings will be observed using all power functions to show this patient the impact of using the power functions (i.e., biofeedback).

Documentation and Communication with the Team on Findings

Education and recommendations include smoking cessation, nutrition, bed positioning, method and frequency of pressure reliefs, encourage working with nursing on bowel and bladder management, and consider counseling for managing mental health needs. The SWM team will review care of the cushion and follow up with more education once his new PWC and seating system arrive. Documentation of all of these topics will be sent back to the wound care medical team and discuss the timing of future seating and mobility clinic visits for follow-up pressure mapping or adjustments are needed. If surgery is recommended, pressure mapping before surgery and after surgery when stable would ensure better outcomes and follow-up. The expertise of the SWM clinician addressing the problems of his postural changes, need for new mobility equipment, assessing his issues with microclimate, and his current functional level allowed a more comprehensive approach and feedback to the medical team on how to improve his overall health and plan of care going forward.

SUMMARY

Traditionally wound care professionals have considered WC seating interventions and evaluations as preventative measures for skin injuries. Today however, SWM clinicians have the expertise and ability to serve as a crucial member of the wound care team. Evaluation of the entire seating system, not just the cushion and pressure mapping, is vital to providing comprehensive recommendations. WC users with or without skin injuries can be referred to an SWM clinic through multiple routes. As a part of the multidisciplinary team, the comprehensive SWM clinician can serve as a lifelong resource for the treatment and prevention of skin injuries as well as for maximizing functional mobility and independence.

CLINICS CARE POINTS

- Consider the 24 hour function and position of someone dealing with pressure injury.
- For a wheelchair user, the cause of the pressure injury may not be the cushion.
- Pressure mapping is a tool to help determine appropriate cushions but does not measure other risk factors such as shear, moisture and trauma from functional activities.
- Pressure mapping can be used as biofeedback and education for teaching pressure relief techniques to patients.

REFERENCES

1. Kottner J, Cuddigan J, Carville K, et al. Prevention and treatment of pressure ulcers/injuries: The protocol for the second update of the international Clinical Practice Guideline 2019. J Tissue Viability 2019;28(2):51–8.
2. Moore KD, Hardin A, VanHoose L, et al. Current wound care education in entry-level doctor of physical therapy curricula. Adv Skin Wound Care 2020;33(1): 47–52.
3. RESNA Wheelchair Service Provision Guide, Rehabilitation Engineering and Assistive Technology Society of North America; Published January 26, 2011; Accessed September 2021.
4. Centers for Medicare and Medicaid (CMS). DMEPOS Quality Standards. 2020. Available at: https://www.cms.gov/Outreach-and-Education/Medicare-Learning-Network-MLN/MLNProducts/DMEPOSQuality/DMEPOSQualBooklet-905709. html. Accessed October 20, 2021.
5. APTA analysis: the value of physical therapy in wound care. American Physical Therapy Association website; 2020. Available at: https://www.apta.org/article/ 2020/10/30/analysis-value-physical -therapy-wound-care. Accessed October 10, 2021.
6. Shi C, Dumville JC, Cullum N. Support surfaces for pressure ulcer prevention: a network meta-analysis. PLoS One 2018;13(2):e0192707.
7. Kennedy P, Berry C, Coggrave M, et al. The effect of a specialist seating assessment clinic on the skin management of individuals with spinal cord injury. J Tissue Viability 2003;13(3):122–5.
8. Bhattacharya S, Mishra RK. Pressure ulcers: Current understanding and newer modalities of treatment. Indian J Plast Surg 2015;48(1):4–16.
9. International review: pressure ulcer prevention: pressure, shear, friction and microclimate in context. London: Wounds International; 2010.
10. Gefen A, Weihs D. Cytoskeleton and plasma-membrane damage resulting from exposure to sustained deformations: a review of the mechanobiology of chronic wounds. Med Eng Phys 2016;38(9):828–33.
11. Capuano P, Capasso G. Il ruolo del pH intracellulare nella regolazione della funzione cellulare [The importance of intracellular pH in the regulation of cell function]. G Ital Nefrol 2003;20(2):139–50.
12. Lagadic-Gossmann D, Huc L, Lecureur V. Alterations of intracellular pH homeostasis in apoptosis: origins and roles. Cell Death Differ 2004;11(9):953–61.
13. International Organization for Standardization. Wheelchair seating — Part 9: Clinical interface pressure mapping guidelines for seating. ISO/TR 16840-9:2015 Published 2015. Accessed October 5, 2021.

14. Stinson M, Crawford S. Wheelchair seating and pressure mapping. In: Söderback I, editor. International handbook of occupational therapy interventions. 2nd edition. New York: Springer; 2015. p. 221–31.
15. Lange ML, Minkel J. Seating and wheeled mobility: a clinical resource guide. Thorofare, NJ: Slack Incorporated; 2018.
16. Rice I. Manual wheelchair propulsion biomechanics and upper limb pain, exploring injury mechanisms and preventive strategies. Directions 2015;3:41–3.
17. Cooper R. Proper set-up and training to optimize self-propulsion of manual wheelchairs. Directions 2015;3:44–8.
18. Waugh K, Crane B, Taylor S, et al. A clinical application guide to standardized wheelchair seating measures of the body and seating support surface. Revised Edition. Denver, CO: The Regents of University of Colorado, Assistive Technology Partners; 2013.
19. Waugh K, Crane B, Taylor S, et al. Glossary of wheelchair terms and definitions. Version 1.0. Denver, CO: The Regents of University of Colorado; 2013. Assistive Technology Partners.
20. Bonifant H, Holloway S. A review of the effects of ageing on skin integrity and wound healing. Br J Community Nurs 2019;24(Sup3):S28–33.

APPENDIX 1: PRESSURE MAP VALUE

Pressure Map Value	Definition and Interpretation
Dispersion index (%)	The sum of pressure distributed over a region (e.g. the IT and the sacral-coccygeal region) divided by the sum of pressure readings over the entire sensor mat, expressed as a percentage. A value of 50% or more is indicative of a potential risk of skin trauma.
Peak pressure index (PPI)	The average of the highest recorded pressure values within a 9–10 cm² area (the contact area of an IT). PPI is a better comparative benchmark than average seat pressures.
Sensing Area (in²)	The area of the mat the consumer is resting on which is displaying above the minimum setting, e.g., 5 mm Hg. Generally, a larger sensing or contact area is preferred, which means the area of support has increased.
Coefficient of Variation (CoV, %)	The coefficient of variation shows how evenly the pressure is distributed across a support surface. It is expressed as a percentage and is normally the inverse of the sensing area. It is better to have a lower CoV value but ensure comparison to the pressure map readings; you may have a low CoV but still have a high localized force somewhere in the seat surface.
Gradient	The gradient identifies areas of the skin that may be affected by shear forces and is expressed as mm Hg/cm. Areas of fastest change in pressure over the surface of the seat are displayed as hotter colors. It is felt that where pressures change quickly from one location to another there is a risk of shear occurring to the tissue.

Establishing a Comprehensive Wound Care Team and Program

Scott Schubert, MD[a],*, George Marzloff, MD[a],
Stephanie Ryder, MD[a], Kaila Ott, MS, ATP[a],
Jennifer Hutton, MS, RN, CNS, CWCN, CRRN[a],
Mallory Becker, RN, BSN, CWCN, CRRN[b]

KEYWORDS

- Physician • Therapist • Psychology • Nursing • Surgery • Myocutaneous flap
- Debridement • Colostomy

KEY POINTS

- A comprehensive, interdisciplinary team is the ideal approach to wound management.
- Generally led by a rehabilitation physician, the team involves wound care nurses, surgeons, physical and occupational therapists, dieticians, psychologists, infectious diseases physicians, a nursing team, and patients and caregivers.
- A case study describes the clinical course from development of pressure injury through the healing process, highlighting the role each team member provides to the patient.

INTRODUCTION

Once a wound or pressure injury has developed, it presents a significant potential for morbidity and mortality. Vascular wounds and diabetic wounds can lead to potential limb loss, systemic infection, or falls leading to further injury. Development of a pressure injury during acute care hospitalization or during rehabilitation admission can delay or alter the ultimate potential for functional improvement.[1] Furthermore, the cost of effective wound management is substantial.[2–4] To maximize the outcome for the patient and to most efficiently use medical resources, having a comprehensive interdisciplinary team is the ideal approach to wound management (**Fig. 1**). The composition of this team may vary depending on the nature of the wound (ie, vascular, diabetic, or pressure) and may vary depending on the severity of the wound or comorbidities.

Once a comprehensive wound care team has been established, frequent interdisciplinary rounding facilitates open communication, complex case planning, and

[a] Rocky Mountain Regional VA Medical Center, 1700 North Wheeling Street (K1-11SC), Aurora, CO 80045, USA; [b] Robley Rex VA Medical Center, Fort Knox CBOC, Fort Knox, KY 40121, USA
* Corresponding author.
E-mail address: scott.schubert2@va.gov

Phys Med Rehabil Clin N Am 33 (2022) 805–810
https://doi.org/10.1016/j.pmr.2022.06.006
1047-9651/22/Published by Elsevier Inc.

pmr.theclinics.com

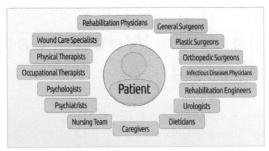

Fig. 1. Interdisciplinary team model to patient-centered wound care management. Many disciplines contribute to the patient's wound healing process.

efficiency of care. Frequent interdisciplinary meetings can help to identify patients for intervention, coordinate interventions by multiple team members, and improve overall outcomes for the patient.

Because of the complexity of wound management and overlapping expertise and training, the roles of specific wound care team members may vary by location, but the discussion in this article provides a rough outline for consideration when creating an interdisciplinary wound care program or team.

CARE SETTINGS

Because of the complex and potentially chronic nature of wounds and pressure injuries, an ideal wound care team bridges the gap between cares provided in the home, outpatient clinic–based wound care, and inpatient complex wound management.

For initial evaluation or maintenance care for minor chronic wounds, an outpatient clinic setting is ideal to allow frequent rechecks while maintaining patient autonomy. This also minimizes the potential for hospital-acquired infections and provides a more cost-effective option. The outpatient wound clinic should be able to provide clinical wound evaluation, basic laboratory evaluation, dressing management, and consultation with specialties.

Wounds that are severe on first presentation, show signs of infection, or that require surgical intervention may justify an inpatient admission for complex management. The inpatient setting can allow for specialized wound evaluation including advanced imaging; invasive testing, such as bone or tissue biopsy; 24-hour monitoring; and consultative services from critical care teams.

Additionally, a home care team is an important part of the team to assist with routine dressing changes, evaluate living situations and home surfaces, and alert the outpatient/inpatient team of early clinical changes.

REHABILITATION PHYSICIANS

A rehabilitation physician who is trained in wound management can serve as team leader. Physical medicine and rehabilitation residency training highlights the interdisciplinary approach to health care, making the rehabilitation physician uniquely suited to coordination of care among a variety of unique specialties. Additionally this residency training provides a background knowledge of amputation medicine, wound care, and management of patients at high risk for pressure injury following neurotrauma.

The rehabilitation physician should be familiar with basic wound dressing options, selective sharp debridement, and medical comorbidities that place an individual at higher risk for skin injury, such as spinal cord injury, brain injury, stroke, or neuromuscular dysfunction. The rehabilitation physician is also able to educate the patient and create a treatment plan that addresses other common rehabilitation issues, such as spasticity, neurogenic bowel management, and neurogenic bladder management that may either predispose a patient to wounds or delay wound healing and prevent closure when a wound has already occurred.

The rehabilitation physician can also serve as the director and coordinator for referrals to other specialists on the wound care team as indicated during the healing process.

CERTIFIED WOUND CARE SPECIALISTS

Certified wound care nurses or therapists with wound care certification provide expertise in specialty conservative wound management and are frequently the first team member to evaluate a patient referred with a new wound. They can provide consultation for specialty wound dressings; coordinate specialty therapies, such as ultrasonic mist treatment; and provide education to the patient, family, and general nursing team about dressing management. They often are the primary clinical caregiver for outpatient wound care clinics or the first point of contact for clinical teams on inpatient hospital units. Nurses with ostomy training assist patients who elect to undergo diverting colostomy (discussed in the next section).

SURGEONS

It is often necessary to involve one or more surgical specialties to help manage a complex wound optimally.

General surgery can provide more extensive tissue debridement beyond the selective sharp debridement offered by the rehabilitation physician. Depending on wound location and ability to maintain continence, general surgery may provide options for colostomy creation to optimize the potential for wound healing.

If a pressure injury is severe and cannot be adequately healed by conservative measures, a plastic or reconstructive surgeon may need to evaluate the patient to consider a flap procedure to mobilize healthy tissue to cover an area of nonviable wound tissue.

If there is extensive bony involvement or signs of deep osteomyelitis in the wound area, the orthopedic surgical service should be consulted to evaluate the wound. They may also be able to obtain deep bone biopsy specimens for evaluation by pathology, which can influence antibiotic treatment and definitive surgical closure timing.

Urology may need to be involved if urine incontinence is contributing to wound development or if the wound has caused erosion into urinary tract structures. Depending on the extent of the issue, the urology team may need to create a urologic diversion, such as placement of a suprapubic catheter.

Vascular surgery may need to intervene if there is decreased blood flow or tissue oxygenation that prevents the healing of an extremity wound. This may include surgical or minimally invasive procedures to improve blood flow to the affected site. In many centers, vascular surgery may coordinate the need for limb amputation if a wound has caused a limb to be nonviable.

PHYSICAL THERAPISTS, OCCUPATIONAL THERAPISTS, AND REHABILITATION ENGINEERS

In addition to potentially being certified in wound management, physical and occupational therapists may provide specialized expertise on adaptive equipment or specialty surfaces that may help improve the potential of wound healing by offloading pressure or preventing shearing. They may have movement strategies, assistive devices, or custom equipment modifications that would allow a patient to remain independent and active while working to heal their wound. Therapists can provide a comprehensive assessment of support surfaces, seating surfaces, bathroom equipment, and transfers, using manual methods or pressure mapping technology, to identify any contributors to pressure injury development in hopes of preventing repeat wounds in the future. Rehabilitation engineers provide technical expertise to manage the interface between technology and patient use and provide support to therapists for interpretation of data.

DIETICIANS

Because of the multifactorial nature of wounds and pressure injuries, a specialized registered dietician can provide significant support to the patient by maximizing nutritional status to facilitate wound healing. For instance, healthy protein and increased albumin levels can aid in tissue healing and decrease fluid extravasation. For venous stasis wounds, a dietician may have advice to improve fluid management to minimize edema. For diabetic wounds, improved control of hemoglobin A_{1c} by dietary measures may decrease the potential for progression of diabetic neuropathy.

PSYCHOLOGISTS AND PSYCHIATRISTS

A behavioral health team (eg, psychology or psychiatry) is a strong addition to a wound care team when behavioral components may be exacerbating a wound or if the wound itself creates increasing feelings of depression and isolation. For severe pressure injuries, often a period of prolonged bedrest may be necessary to optimize wound healing, and as a result of this, feelings of isolation and depression can easily arise. For severe wounds where amputation of wounds may become necessary, the behavioral health team can work with the patient to develop coping strategies and improve the outlook for recovery following surgery.

INFECTIOUS DISEASES PHYSICIANS

Chronic open wounds disrupt the protective barrier between the external environment and internal structures. As a result of the disruption of the epithelium, patients can develop localized or systemic infections. Often individuals with chronic wounds have frequent or prolonged hospitalizations, which can expose them to drug-resistant organisms. With this potential for acute or chronic infections, complex antibiotic or antifungal treatment plans may be necessary to aid in wound healing, and so consultation with an experienced infectious disease team is beneficial for improving treatment of the infection and minimizing risks for development of further resistance in an organism.

NURSING TEAM

Registered nurses and certified nursing assistants provide support in outpatient and inpatient settings. For outpatient clinics, nursing staff assists with transfers for wound assessment, dressing changes, and patient education, particularly if the patient is struggling with bowel or bladder incontinence that is contributing to wound persistence. In inpatient settings, the nursing team is critical to ensure proper turns and offloading of the wound. Ideally, patients with wounds are managed bedside by nursing staff who have received specific training on these positioning techniques to prevent harmful pressure, shear, or pulling on the wound. The nursing team also provides wound assessments and dressing changes between evaluations by wound care nurses, rehabilitation physicians, surgical teams, and other specialists.

PATIENTS AND CAREGIVERS

In addition to a strong multidisciplinary clinical team, it is crucial to have participation from the patient and caregivers (if available) in the development of an effective wound care program. Without buy-in from the patient, even the most ideal wound care plan can easily fail. Careful compliance to treatment recommendations and care plans is essential to improve tissue quality and allow for healing to occur. Even surgical interventions fail if the patient is not compliant with postoperative recommendations.

Caregivers can also provide physical and emotional support to help ensure the success of a wound management strategy. This can range from assistance with dressing changes between visits with the wound team, transportation to and from appointments, and at times physical caregiving and support for activities of daily living during the recovery process. Additionally, a poorly supportive caregiver or acquaintance may have a negative behavioral influence that could potentiate tissue damage. For example, a significant other who continues to smoke inside the home may make nicotine cessation difficult for a patient with severe peripheral arterial disease.

CASE STUDY

The following is a narrative of a common scenario of wound care management at our center intended to show the role each discipline plays through the full course of a patient's care. Rafael is a 73-year-old man with chronic complete tetraplegia who has had fairly healthy skin for decades since his spinal cord injury but has had a decline in function recently and developed a pressure injury over the left ischial tuberosity. He suspects it developed during a 3-day lapse in home care support. His spouse reports frequent involuntary bowel movements despite a daily bowel program and is concerned about the wound hygiene. He presented to our wound care clinic with a stage 4 pressure injury and continued to follow up for 8 weeks, but the wound's volume did not improve significantly during that time. MRI showed evidence suggestive of ischial osteomyelitis, which may be interfering with wound healing. We discussed his case at an interdisciplinary team meeting and recommended inpatient admission for definitive treatment.

Rafael was admitted under a rehabilitation physician and all relevant disciplines were consulted. The registered dietician worked to optimize his nutrition to facilitate healing and collagen synthesis. Physical and occupational therapists evaluated his power wheelchair with pressure mapping to evaluate causes of increased pressure on the ischium. Orthopedic surgeons performed a deep bone biopsy, and the infectious disease team started an intravenous antibiotic based on the bone culture results. The general surgeons performed a diverting colostomy early in the admission to minimize stool contamination in the wound. Inpatient wound care nurses assessed the wound and devised a treatment plan to optimize the wound for surgery including selection of specialty surface mattress.

A rehabilitation psychologist worked with the patient on coping with the long-term stay at the hospital. After the antibiotic course was complete, the plastic surgeons performed a myocutaneous flap closure. Wound care nurses continued to monitor the surgical site postoperatively and guided staff for best positioning for flat (or close to flat) bedrest. Rafael recovered for several weeks on the spinal cord injury unit on bed rest restriction with diligent offloading of the flap site and proper turn technique to prevent incisional shearing provided by rehabilitation nurses and certified nursing assistants. His spouse participated in caregiver training with therapists, and the patient was able to return home with a new seat cushion on his power wheelchair. His wound was monitored by outpatient wound care nurses for skin checks and ongoing education.

Additionally, a social worker could be a helpful addition to the wound care team to assist with coordinating community resources because pressure injuries are challenging from a care coordination standpoint.

SUMMARY

Wounds often require complex management, necessitating input from numerous disciplines to successfully treat. This management functions best for the patient when all members of the team are in regular discussion regarding the wound care plan, providing more efficient and timelier patient-centered care.

CLINICS CARE POINTS

- The wound care team comprises staff from many disciplines necessary for optimal wound healing and to diminish the rate of recurrence.
- The patient must be agreeable to the wound care plan for the wound care to be successful. Behavioral health teams can assist with developing coping strategies for the patient.
- The precise team structure for each patient depends on wound severity and type. Interdisciplinary rounding should be frequent to facilitate open communication, case planning, and efficient patient care.

DISCLOSURE

None of the authors has any financial disclosures to report, and they do not have any funding sources to report.

REFERENCES

1. Richard-Denis A, Feldman D, Thompson C, et al. Prediction of functional recovery six months following traumatic spinal cord injury during acute care hospitalization. J Spinal Cord Med 2018;41(3):309–17.
2. Phillips CJ, Humphreys I, Fletcher J, et al. Estimating the costs associated with the management of patients with chronic wounds using linked routine data: costs of wounds using routine data. Int Wound J 2016;13(6):1193–7.
3. Stroupe K, Manheim L, Evans C, et al. Cost of treating pressure ulcers for veterans with spinal cord injury. Top Spinal Cord Inj Rehabil 2011;16(4):62–73.
4. Brem H, Maggi J, Nierman D, et al. High cost of stage IV pressure ulcers. Am J Surg 2010;200(4):473–7.

Nutrition and Wound Care

Nancy Munoz, DCN, MHA, RDN, FAND[a],*, Mary Litchford, PhD, RDN, LD[b],
Emanuele Cereda, MD, PhD[c]

KEYWORDS

- Nutrition • Pressure injuries • Nutrition guidelines • Malnutrition
- Oral nutrition supplement • Nutrition assessment • Nutrition screening • Wounds

KEY POINTS

- Inadequate nutrient intake unravels a series of chemical reactions in the body that impacts wound healing.
- The EPUAP/NPUAP/PPPIA International Clinical Practice Guideline recommends that nutritional screen be completed for individuals at risk for developing pressure injuries.
- Individuals identified at nutritional risk for malnutrition or with actual malnutrition should be referred to the RDN for an in-depth nutrition assessment.
- All phases of wound healing require additional energy, protein, and micronutrient intake to promote healing.
- The presence of chronic conditions is a risk factor for the development of pressure injuries.
- Nutritional or hydration support should be administered for the purpose of addressing desired and achievable outcomes.

INTRODUCTION

Nutrition is an important component of health and well-being. A compromised nutritional status has been linked to increased risk for wound development, difficulty managing, and decreased wound healing rate. Malnutrition contributes to an immunocompromised system, reduced collagen synthesis, and diminished tensile strength during the wound healing process. Thus, assessment and optimization of nutritional status should be incorporated as part of a comprehensive treatment plan for individuals with wounds. This article reviews the role of nutrition in wound prevention, management, and treatment.

[a] University of Massachusetts, Southern Nevada VA Healthcare System, 7041 Solana Ridge Drive, North Las Vegas, NV 89084, USA; [b] CASE Software & Books, 3912 Battleground Avenue, Suite 112 #175, Greensboro, NC 27410, USA; [c] UOC Dietetica e Nutrizione Clinica, Fondazione IRCCS Policlinico San Matteo, Viale Golgi 1927100, Pavia, Italy
* Corresponding author.
E-mail address: Dr.NMunozRD@outlook.com

Phys Med Rehabil Clin N Am 33 (2022) 811–822
https://doi.org/10.1016/j.pmr.2022.06.007
1047-9651/22/Published by Elsevier Inc.

IMPACT OF MALNUTRITION ON WOUND DEVELOPMENT, MANAGEMENT, AND HEALING

The World Health Organization defines malnutrition as deficiency, excess, and imbalance in an individual's caloric and/or nutrient intake.[1] Malnutrition encompasses three distinct conditions: (1) undernutrition, (2) micronutrient-related malnutrition, and (3) overweight. **Table 1** defines the three conditions involved in malnutrition.

Limited data are available defining actual prevalence of malnutrition and nutritional risk in the acute care setting. Survey results from the Nutrition Day survey reports that one in three patients admitted to the acute care setting are at risk for malnutrition.[2] Worldwide, malnutrition affects 30% to 50% of hospitalized patients.[3–6]

The wound healing process puts the body in an anabolic state that demands specific nutrient intake and proper hydration to support physiologic activities. Inadequate nutrient intake unravels a series of chemical reactions in the body that impacts wound healing. Initially, the body uses the glycogen stored in the liver to support essential cellular functions. Continued nutrient deprivation increases the body's metabolic rate and increases cortisol levels. This facilitates the mobilization of amino acids from the body's protein stores to support hepatic gluconeogenesis to supply the body with glucose (**Fig. 1**).[7,8]

The inflammatory response process increases inflammatory cytokines and decreases negative acute phase reactant protein, such as albumin and prealbumin. Continued nutrient deficit forces the body to metabolize fat as a source of energy while sparing the breakdown of muscle tissue and produces weight loss.[7] Decreased fat stores can contribute to increased pressure on bony prominences, thus increasing the risk for the development of pressure injuries (PIs).

Once the fat stores are depleted, with continued nutrient deficiency, the body uses skeletal muscle for energy, thus producing rapid weight loss and declining muscle mass. Malnutrition contributes to a compromised immune system and decreased muscle function and strength impacts mobility, activities of daily living specific to food preparation and eating, and delays wound healing.[9,10]

Nutritional Screening

The presence of a poor nutritional status has been associated with increased risk for developing PIs.[11,12] Timely detection of patients who are at risk of developing PIs is an essential component of any prevention strategy. The EPUAP/NPUAP/PPPIA International Clinical Practice Guideline recommends that nutritional screen be completed for individuals at risk for developing PIs.[13] Patients identified at risk or with actual

Table 1	
Conditions involved in malnutrition	
Condition	**Definition**
Undernutrition	Involves wasting, stunting, underweight, and deficiencies in vitamin and minerals
Micronutrient-related malnutrition	Inadequate intake of vitamin and minerals
Overweight	This is an imbalance between energy intake and energy expenditure with excessive fat accumulation and inadequate micronutrient intake

Data from World Health Organization. Malnutrition. 2021. https://www.who.int/en/news-room/fact-sheets/detail/malnutrition. Accessed 7/23/2021.

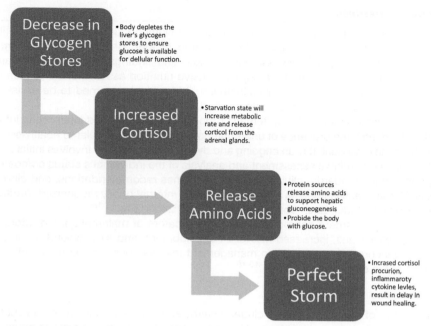

Fig. 1. Malnutrition and wound healing. (*Data from* Heimburger DC. Malnutrition and nutritional assessment. *in Fauci AS et al, editors: Harrison's principles of internal medicine, ed 17, New York, 2008, McGraw-Hill* 2008. Rote NS. Innate Immunity: Inflammation and wound healing. *in: Huether SE, Mc- Cance KL understanding pathophysiology 5th ed St Louis, MO: Elsevier:118-141.* 2012.)

malnutrition should be referred to the registered dietitian/nutritionist (RDN) for the completion of an in-depth nutrition assessment. Patients admitted to health care facilities should be screened for malnutrition on admission and rescreened with changes in conditions.

Any member of the interprofessional team that has been deemed competent can conduct a nutrition screen.[14] Common screening parameters include unintended weight loss, low body mass index, loss of muscle and subcutaneous mass, decreased food intake, localized or generalized fluid accumulation, and decreased functional status.[5] A validated screening tool should be used to assign risk level. Laboratory data are not used in traditional nutrition screens. Serum proteins, such as albumin and prealbumin, are not considered sensitive markers of an individual's nutritional status. Protein intake is not associated with changes in albumin and prealbumin.[14] The validated screening tool must be quick and easy to use, reliable, economic, of low risk to the individual being screened, and suitable for the population being screened and care setting.[15]

There are several nutrition screening tools that have been validated for identifying nutritional risk. These include the Mini Nutritional Assessment, Malnutrition Universal Screening Tool, Nutrition Risk Screening 2002, and the Short Nutritional Assessment Questionnaire. The Mini Nutritional Assessment has been validated for use with older adults with PI and multiple comorbidities.[16] The Malnutrition Universal Screening Tool and the Nutrition Risk Screening 2002 is used in acute, long-term, and community settings.[17] For adults in acute and residential care the Short Nutritional Assessment Questionnaire tool has been deemed a valid and reliable screening tool.[17]

Nutrition Assessment

A comprehensive nutrition assessment using the Nutrition Care Process model includes client history, food- and nutrition-related history, physical measurements, nutrition-focused physical assessment findings, and findings from laboratory and medical tests. The purpose of the comprehensive nutrition assessment is to identify the presence of undernutrition or malnutrition.[18] Individuals deemed to be at risk of PIs are often undernourished or malnourished.[13,15]

Nutrition assessment is the systematic process of collecting and interpreting information to identify the presence of undernutrition- or malnutrition-related health issues that affect an individual. It is an ongoing and dynamic process that involves initial data collection and continual assessment and analysis of the individual's status compared with accepted standards, clinical practice guidelines recommendations, and clinical goals. Nutrition assessment is a component of the internationally recognized Nutrition Care Process Model. Each component is summarized in **Fig. 2**.[18]

Nutrition assessment components identify indicators of malnutrition, indicators of nutrient deficiencies, increased risk for PI development, and slow wound healing. It is vital to incorporate the nutrition management interventions for chronic conditions as part of the skin health program.[13,15]

Nutrients and Wound Healing

The science of wound care has included healthy eating as an essential ingredient for healing wounds since ancient times. However, understanding the role of key nutrients in the complex process of wound healing was not recognized until the twentieth century. All nutrients work synergistically to maintain the body and promote wound healing. No single nutrient stands alone as the sole substrate to replace devitalized tissue with healthy tissue.[19] The most rigorous literature review on the role of nutrition and wound healing is International Clinical Practice Guideline on the Prevention and Treatment of Pressure Injuries.[13] Emerging evidence supports the benefits of higher protein and energy requirements for other types of wounds.[20,21] Malnutrition is a detrimental factor in wound healing of ischemic ulceration, peripheral arterial disease–related

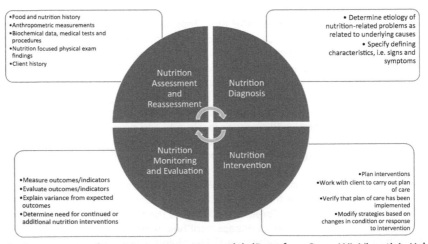

Fig. 2. Components of nutrition care process model. (*Data from* Swan WI, Vivanti A, Hakel-Smith NA, et al. Nutrition Care Process and Model Update: Toward Realizing People-Centered Care and Outcomes Management. *J Acad Nutr Diet.* 2017;117(12). doi: 10.1016/j.jand.2017.07.015.)

wounds, and diabetic foot ulcers.[20–23] Management of chronic conditions associated with wounds must include medical nutrition therapy to optimize wound healing potential.[19] To date there are no published international clinical practice guidelines with nutrition recommendations for other types of wounds.

All phases of wound healing require additional energy and protein intake to promote healing. The International Clinical Practice Guideline recommends individualized assessment for energy and protein requirements based on underlying medical conditions and level of activity. Indirect calorimetry is the most precise approach, but often only available in selected health care settings. The International Clinical Practice Guideline recommendations specify 30 to 35 kcal/kg body weight for adults with a PI who are malnourished or at risk of malnutrition.[13] Malnourished individuals who have unplanned weight loss may require higher energy intakes. Individuals in negative energy balance have higher protein requirements because protein can be used for energy when energy intakes are chronically low.[24]

The International Clinical Practice Guideline recommendations specify 1.25 to 1.5 g/protein/kg body weight for adults with a PI who are malnourished and are at risk of malnutrition.[13] Achieving the recommended protein requirements may be challenging. The National Health and Nutrition Examination Survey data demonstrate a linear decrease in total protein intake in males and females after age 60.[25] Wakimoto and Block[26] compared protein intake of healthy with sick adults. More than 30% of sick men and 25% of sick women aged 65 to 74 did not consume estimated protein needs. More than 40% of sick men and more than 35% of sick women aged 75 and older did not consume estimated protein needs. Older adults are the most likely segment of the population to get sick from a poor diet.[25]

In addition, each phase of wound healing has unique micronutrient requirements. The current research on the specific requirements for individual micronutrients for wound healing has not advanced to specific recommended allowances. Individual nutrient supplementation is not recommended unless specific nutrient deficiencies are suspected or confirmed.[13] Individuals consuming highly restrictive diets or who have low nutrient intakes may benefit from high-potency multiple vitamins with minerals unless contraindicated. Recommendations for vitamin mineral supplementation is based on individualized assessment. **Table 2** identifies key nutrients involved in each phase of wound healing[19,27] and **Table 3** includes food sources of key nutrients involved in wound healing.[19]

IMPACT OF CHRONIC DISEASE ON NUTRITION AND WOUND HEALING

Some of the most common chronic conditions are risk factors for compromised nutritional status and wound development. These include diabetes mellitus (DM) and impaired glucose tolerance (prediabetes), heart failure, atrial fibrillation, chronic obstructive pulmonary disease (COPD), renal insufficiency, anemia, and dementia, to name a few.

Neuropathy and vasculopathy are comorbidities associated with diabetes that increase the risk factor for the development of wounds.[28] DM is often linked with the development of peripheral artery disease. Peripheral artery disease in the presence of diabetic neuropathy can increase the risk of nonhealing wounds and limb loss in individuals with DM.[29,30] Uncontrolled hyperglycemia can also interfere with wound healing. High glucose levels cause the cell walls to become stiff and rigid reducing the blood flow through the small vessels found at the surface of the wound. High glucose levels also interfere with the hemoglobin release of oxygen, thus reducing the availability of oxygen and nutrients in the wound site.[31]

Table 2
Nutrients required for each phase of wound healing[19,27]

Phase of Wound Healing	Key Nutrients
Hemostasis	Protein Energy Vitamin K Ascorbic acid
Inflammation	Protein Energy B-complex vitamins Ascorbic acid
Proliferation	Protein Energy Iron Zinc Copper Ascorbic acid Vitamin A Folate B-complex vitamins
Maturation	Protein Energy Vitamin A Ascorbic acid

Data from Litchford M. Nutrition & Pressure Injuries. *Greensboro, NC CASE Software.* 2020. Mills JL, Sr., Conte MS, Armstrong DG, et al. The Society for Vascular Surgery Lower Extremity Threatened Limb Classification System: risk stratification based on wound, ischemia, and foot infection (WIfI). *J Vasc Surg.* 2014;59(1):220-234.e221-222.

Oxygen is required for all stages of wound healing, thus any condition that is associated with a low tissue oxygen tension may increase the risk for developing PIs. These include: heart failure, atrial fibrillation, myocardial infarction, and COPD.[31]

Individuals who have chronic kidney disease or end-stage renal disease on hemodialysis suffer from a uremic state that decelerates different organ systems including

Table 3
Food sources of key nutrients required for wound healing

Nutrient	Food Sources
Protein	Meat, fish, poultry, pulses (dried beans and peas), dairy products, soy foods
B-complex vitamins	Fortified grains, pasta, milk, poultry, fish, eggs, legumes
Folate	Fortified grains, lima, lentil and garbanzo beans, leafy green vegetables
Vitamin A	Sweet potatoes, carrots, leafy green vegetables
Ascorbic acid	Citrus fruits, guavas, berries, broccoli, tomatoes
Vitamin K	Broccoli, dark green leafy vegetables
Iron	Meat, poultry, eggs, fortified grains, pulses (dried beans and peas)
Copper	Organ meats, fish, cashews, sunflower seeds, fortified grains
Zinc	Red meat, oysters, almonds, peanuts, fortified grains

Data from Litchford M. Nutrition & Pressure Injuries. *Greensboro, NC CASE Software.* 2020.

the gastrointestinal tract. These patients usually experience decreased appetite (anorexia) and overall decreased nutrient intake.[32]

Anemia can diminish adequate transfer of nutrients and oxygen to promote tissue healing. Anemia comes in several forms, but the most common is the type linked to iron deficiency. In patients with iron deficiency, there is reduced production of hemoglobin. This translates into decreased oxygen circulating from the lungs into tissues throughout the body. Iron deficiency also contributes to poor appetite and cravings for substances with no nutritional value, such as dirt, starch, and ice.[33]

Individuals with dementia or psychiatric disorders regularly suffer from agitation and confusion. Many exhibit feeding difficulties and require assistance at meals. Care for these patients is challenging because with disease progression they do not recognize food, and/or sensations of hunger and thirst. This can affect their overall nutritional status resulting in increased risk for malnutrition and reduced healing rate.[34]

NUTRITION INTERVENTIONS AND WOUND HEALING

Nutrition and hydration are essential for life and problems arise when a person cannot cope with these requirements in part or at all. Nutrition is a transversal science and it is well accepted that good nutrition is associated with better prognosis in many diseases. This statement is substantially supported by the numerous guidelines produced for the purpose of optimizing nutritional management from a multidisciplinary perspective.[35] The creation of interprofessional teams should be therefore on the agenda of clinicians and resource allocators.

Screening positive for nutritional risk is now considered for prompt interventions and designing tailored nutritional care plans, regardless of but taking into account the clinical condition and the setting of care.[36] It is unquestionable that good nutrition sustains tissue viability and promotes the healing process. Nonetheless, wounds are likely responsible for the loss of nutrients and an increase of energy needs.[37] Evidence of efficacy of interventions is not substantial for all the types of wounds but strong recommendations do exist for patients suffering from or at risk of developing PIs.[13] Indeed, lack of nutrients is more relevant than their excess, although body weight loss may be useful in patients with venous leg ulcers and optimal glucose control is mandatory for improving the outcome of diabetic ulcers. Therefore, reaching energy goals in patients with wounds is important.

The nutrition care plan is based on the information gathered in the nutrition assessment, particularly data on protein-calorie intake, energy needs associated also with disease burden, and overall capacity of the patient to satisfy them with or without the aid of a caregiver. But prescription is only the first step. Routine or periodic monitoring of the care plan is the most important component of the nutrition care process. Interventions must be adjusted with any change in conditions and when progress toward the desired outcome is not achieved.

How to Evaluate Oral Intake

Taking into account that wounds are closely linked to malnutrition, a formal quantification of food intake is an invaluable step in nutritional assessment. Therefore, this evaluation should rely on the use of quantitative or semiquantitative tools, such as multiple 24-hour dietary recalls or food intake charts (kept by health care staff or caregivers) or 3- to 7-day food diaries.[14,38] Indeed, all these tools require a higher participation of the patients or caregivers but enable a more precise estimation of protein-calorie and to better guide nutrition specialists in tailoring nutritional care plans. If their use is not feasible because of clinical conditions or logistic difficulties, the use of alternative proxy measures, such as those included in screening tools, should also be recommended.[39,40] Nonetheless, in patients receiving artificial nutrition, quantification should take into account also this source of nutrients.

Strategies to Increase Oral Intake

Optimization of oral diet represents the first-line strategy for every patient still able to consume food intake.[14,38] To this purpose, the role played by the RDN is fundamental. Nutritional counseling is currently a recommended standard of care. It consists of a personalized dietary prescription, including the provision and sample meal plans and recipe suggestions, modeled on and adapted to personal eating patterns and preferences (including cultural/religious ones), taking into account clinical conditions, comorbidities, chewing and swallowing abilities, and nutrition impact symptoms (chewing difficulties, dysphagia, anorexia, dysgeusia, nausea, vomiting, diarrhea, and constipation). Energy density, macronutrients distribution, and texture are therefore tailored to satisfy estimated protein-calorie requirements. If needed, liberalization of dietary restrictions resulting in decreased intake should be considered. Offering assistance with eating and providing a pleasant eating environment could also contribute substantially to improved food intake.

Finally yet importantly, regular consultations by an RDN must be provided on a variable frequency to refine the care plan and depending on patient's conditions, treatment, and goals.

Use of Fortified Foods and Oral Nutritional Supplements

Strategies to increase oral intake with nutritional counseling comprise food fortification and the use of oral nutritional supplements (ONSs). Although the former could be reasonably considered a first-line approach, used to improve the intake of key micronutrients in presence of adequate macronutrients intake, the latter frequently represent a second-step procedure, prescribed when patients are unable to achieve or maintain satisfactory protein-calorie intake (usually <60% of estimated requirements for 2 consecutive weeks) with diet optimization.[14,38] Systematic literature review of randomized clinical trials supports their use because of their good tolerance and their efficacy in improving energy balance and clinical outcomes, especially when higher-energy-density ONSs (1.5–2.4 kcal/mL) are consumed between meals.[41] Indeed, health professionals are advised to weigh their value for the treatment plan also after reviewing the nutrition labeling to balance nutrient adequacy because available products supply different amounts of macronutrients and micronutrients.

The use of fortified food is not evidence-based and could not be formally recommended. However, evidence on the efficacy of ONSs in increasing the rate of healing is consistent and substantiated by different trials. Particularly, there is evidence for recommending specific blends in patients at nutritional risk undergoing major elective surgery and in those suffering from PIs.[13,42]

ONSs enriched in immunonutrients (arginine + nucleotides + ω-3 fatty acids) provided before surgery may help reduce wound infections, anastomotic leakage, and length of stay, whereas the use of high-protein ONSs enriched with arginine, zinc, and antioxidants results in improved healing of PIs.[13,42] However, the efficacy of ONS-based intervention is likely time-dependent. Immunonutrition before surgery should be provided for at least 5 to 7 days, whereas the duration of intervention in patients with PIs should be at least 4 weeks and reasonably up to complete healing. Protein-enriched ONS in at-risk patients may contribute also to prevent the development of PIs.[13,42]

Use of Enteral/Parenteral Nutrition

There is currently limited evidence supporting artificial nutrition for improving healing outcome. However, in individuals who cannot meet their nutrition requirements through oral intake despite previous intervention, the risks and benefits of enteral nutrition (EN; tube feeding) or parenteral nutrition (PN) should be discussed by the interprofessional team and with the patient and/or caregivers (cultural and/or religious values may influence acceptance or refusal), and consistently with the individual's goals of care: improve nutrition status, promote healing, and restore immune function.[13,38]

Artificial nutrition could be either total or integrative (supplemental) and the involvement of a nutrition specialist is mandatory to optimize its provision according to estimated requirements and residual spontaneous food intake. EN is always the preferred route and the first choice if the gastrointestinal tract is functioning, because it helps maintain or improve the immune function. PN should be considered for patients who cannot meet nutrition requirements with EN or refuse it. As applies to ONSs, different commercial formulations are available and their choice and use should be tailored to patient's requirements. Clinicians should also routinely check and confirm that administrations are in line with prescriptions, evaluate tolerance to treatment, and note any adverse reactions.

In surgical patients undergoing elective surgery and in whom postoperative EN is indicated, the use of immunonutrition should be considered to avoid wound-related complications and improve healing outcome. Nonetheless, perioperative fluid administration, which can depend also on PN, should be managed in a state of near-zero balance to avoid insufficient tissue perfusion and complications associated with overload, such as impaired immune function and anastomotic leakage.[42]

Finally, nutrition goals should not take priority over the patient-centered goals and the interdisciplinary team should consider if the patient has the desire and/or capacity to tolerate nutrition support.

NUTRITION CARE AT END OF LIFE

Nutritional or hydration support, as true medical treatments, should be administered for the purpose of addressing desired and achievable outcomes:[15,43,44]

- Prolonging or preserving life
- Enhancing or preserving quality of life (if necessary by accepting a shortening of the time left to live)

Patients receiving palliative care are at high risk of impaired healing because of immobility, serious illness, and worse prognosis and suitable interventions must be implemented on an individual level after appropriate discussion of benefits and harms and taking into account the caregiving context. Indeed, following the "Primum non nocere" principle, potential benefits have to be maximized, while minimizing potential harm because a distinction between beneficence and nonmaleficence still exists. Disproportionate treatments must be avoided because life prolongation should never turn in prolonging of the dying phase. Health care professionals may only suggest interventions, which is realized only if the patient wishes to do so. It is the position of the Academy of Nutrition and Dietetics that "individuals have the right to request or refuse nutrition and hydration as medical treatment" and European Society of Clinical Nutrition and Metabolism states that a "competent patient has the right to refuse a treatment after adequate information even when this refusal would lead to his or her death."[43,44]

SUMMARY

The wound healing process requires proper nutrition and hydration. Risk for or the presence of malnutrition has been linked to increased risk for developing PIs. Adequate nutritional intake and hydration are essential to promote wound healing. Nutrients work synergistically to promote tissue growth and regeneration. No single nutrient stands alone as the sole substrate to replace devitalized tissue with healthy tissue. Management of chronic conditions linked to wounds requires medical nutrition therapy to enhance wound healing potential.

Chronic conditions, such as DM, COPD, anemia, and heart conditions, have an impact on wound development and healing. These conditions must be addressed to maximize the benefit of nutrition interventions.

The nutrition care plan must include individualized interventions designed to address the individual's nutrition diagnosis.

CLINICS CARE POINTS

- Conduct a nutrition screen to identify risk for developing PIs.
- Individuals identified at risk for or with an actual PI should be referred to the RDN for an in-depth nutrition assessment to be conducted.
- In collaboration with the interdisciplinary team, develop a patient-centered care plan.
- Promote the consumption of a healthy diet that meets the individual's nutrient needs.
- When nutritional intake is insufficient to meet the individual's nutritional needs, provide a high-calorie, high-protein ONS between meals.
- Evaluate the need for ONS enriched with arginine, zinc, and antioxidant for individuals with PIs who are at risk for or malnourished to meet their calculated nutritional needs.
- When compatible with the individual's goals, discuss the need for artificial nutrition (EN or PN) for those unable to consume adequate intake.
- Offer palliative/hospice care based on individual's wishes.

DISCLOSURE

No conflict of interest.

REFERENCES

1. World Health Organization. Malnutrition. 2021. Available at: https://www.who.int/en/news-room/fact-sheets/detail/malnutrition. Accessed July 23, 2021.
2. Sauer AC, Goates S, Malone A, et al. Prevalence of malnutrition risk and the impact of nutrition risk on hospital outcomes: results from nutritionday in the U.S. JPEN J Parenter Enteral Nutr 2019;43(7):918–26.
3. Steiber A, Hegazi R, Herrera M, et al. Spotlight on global malnutrition: a continuing challenge in the 21st century. J Acad Nutr Diet 2015;115(8):1335–41.
4. Tappenden K, Quatrara B, Parkhurst M, et al. Critical role of nutrition in improving quality of care: an interdisciplinary call to action to address adult hospital malnutrition. J Acad Nutr Diet 2013;113(9):1219–37.
5. White JV, Guenter P, Jensen G, et al. Consensus statement: Academy of Nutrition and Dietetics and American Society for Parenteral and Enteral Nutrition:

characteristics recommended for the identification and documentation of adult malnutrition (undernutrition). J Parenter Enteral Nutr 2012;36(3):275–83.

6. Cederholm T, Barazzoni R, Austin P, et al. ESPEN guidelines on definitions and terminology of clinical nutrition. Clin Nutr 2017;36(1):49–64.

7. Heimburger DC. Malnutrition and nutritional assessment. In: Fauci AS, et al, editors. Harrison's principles of internal medicine, 17. New York: McGraw-Hill; 2008.

8. Rote NS. Innate immunity: inflammation and wound healing. In: Huether SE, editor. Mc- Cance KL understanding pathophysiology. 5th edition. St Louis, MO: Elsevier; 2012. p. 118–41.

9. Jaffee L, Wu S. The role of nutrition in chronic wound care management. Podiatry Management 2017. Available at: https://podiatrym.com/pdf/2017/11/JaffeWu1117web.pdf. Accessed July 21, 2021.

10. Haydock DA, Hill GL. Impaired wound healing in surgical patients with varying degrees of malnutrition. JPEN J Parenter Enteral Nutr 1986;10(6):550–4.

11. Berlowitz DR, Wilking SV. Risk factors for pressure sores. A comparison of cross-sectional and cohort-derived data. J Am Geriatr Soc 1989;37:1043–50.

12. Pinchcofsky-Devin GD, Kaminski MV. Correlation of pressure sores and nutritional status. J Am Geriatr Soc 1986;34:435–40.

13. Haesler E, editor. European Pressure Ulcer Advisory Panel, National Pressure Injury Advisory Panel and Pan Pacific Pressure Injury Alliance. Prevention and treatment of pressure ulcers/injuries: clinical practice guideline. The International Guideline EPUAP/NPIAP/PPPIA; 2019. p. 94–114.

14. Academy of Nutrition and Dietetics. Nutrition care manual. 2021. Available at: http://www.nutritioncaremanual.org/. Accessed July 26, 2021.

15. Munoz N, Posthauer ME, Cereda E, et al. The role of nutrition for pressure injury prevention and healing: the 2019 International Clinical Practice Guideline recommendations. Adv Skin Wound Care 2020;33(3):123–36.

16. Grattagliano I, Marasciulo L, Paci CMN, et al. The assessment of the nutritional status predicts the long term risk of major events in older individuals. Eur Geriatr Med 2017;8(3):273–4.

17. Poulia KA, Yannakoulia M, Karageorgou D, et al. Evaluation of the efficacy of six nutritional screening tools to predict malnutrition in the elderly. Clin Nutr 2012; 31(3):378–85.

18. Swan WI, Vivanti A, Hakel-Smith NA, et al. Nutrition care process and model update: toward realizing people-centered care and outcomes management. J Acad Nutr Diet 2017;117(12). https://doi.org/10.1016/j.jand.2017.07.015.

19. Litchford M. Nutrition & pressure injuries. Greensboro: NC CASE Software; 2020. p. 77–127.

20. Delaney CL, Smale MK, Miller MD. Nutritional considerations for peripheral arterial disease: a narrative review. Nutrients 2019;11(6):1219.

21. Ye J, Mani R. A systematic review and meta-analysis of nutritional supplementation in chronic lower extremity wounds. Int J Low Extrem Wounds 2016;15(4):296–302.

22. Gau BR, Chen HY, Hung SY, et al. The impact of nutritional status on treatment outcomes of patients with limb-threatening diabetic foot ulcers. J Diabetes Complications 2016;30(1):138–42.

23. Lauwers P, Dirinck E, Van Bouwel S, et al. Malnutrition and its relation with diabetic foot ulcer severity and outcome: a review. Acta Clin Belg 2020;29:1–7.

24. Pellett PL. In: Scrimshaw, editor. Protein-energy interactions. Lausanne, Switzerland: International Dietary Energy Consultative Group (IDECG).; 1992. p. 81–121. Available at: http://www.nzdl.org/cgi-bin/library.cgi?e=d-00000-00—off-0ccgi-00-0——0-10-0—0—0direct-10—4————0-1l-11-en-50—20-

about—00-0-1-00-0-0-11-1-0utfZz-8-00&a=d&c=ccgi&cl=CL3.1&d=HASH45c a5b9c6ad120e289fbc3.8.4.1. Accessed October 1, 2021.

25. Wright JD, Wang CY. Dietary intake of ten key nutrients for public health, US 1999-2000. Advance data from vital and health statistics, 334. Hyattsville, MD: NCHS; 2003. p. 1–4.

26. Wakimoto P, Block G. Dietary intake, dietary patterns and changes with age: an epidemiological perspective. J Gerontol A Biol Sci Med Sci 2001;56(2):65–80.

27. Demling RH. Nutrition, anabolism and the wound healing process. Eplasty 2009; 9:65–94. Available at: http://www.medscape.com/viewarticle/711879. Accessed September 27, 2021.

28. Mills JL, Conte MS, Armstrong DG, et al. The Society for Vascular Surgery Lower Extremity Threatened Limb Classification System: risk stratification based on wound, ischemia, and foot infection (WIfI). J Vasc Surg 2014;59(1):220–34, e221-222.

29. Santilli JD, Santilli SM. Chronic critical limb ischemia: diagnosis, treatment and prognosis. Am Fam Physician 1999;59(7):1899–908.

30. Singh N, Armstrong DG, Lipsky BA. Preventing foot ulcers in patients with diabetes. JAMA 2005;293(2):217–28.

31. Guo S, DiPietro LA. Factors affecting wound healing. J Dent Res 2010;89(3): 219–29. Available at: https://www.ncbi.nlm.nih.gov/pmc/articles/PMC2903966/. Accessed July 26, 21.

32. Maroz N, Simman R. Wound healing in patients with impaired kidney function. J Am Coll Clin Wound Spec 2014;5(1):2–7.

33. Wright JA, Richards T, Srai SKS. The role of iron in the skin and cutaneous wound healing. Front Pharmacol 2014;5:156.

34. Jaul E, Meiron O. Dementia and pressure ulcers: is there a close pathophysiological interrelation? J Alzheimers Dis 2017;56(3):861–6.

35. ESPEN Guidelines and Consensus Papers. ESPEN guidelines and consensus papers. 2021. Available at: https://www.espen.org/guidelines-home/espen-guidelines. Accessed September 25, 2021.

36. Elia M, Zellipour L, Stratton RJ. To screen or not to screen for adult malnutrition? Clin Nutr 2005;24(6):867–84.

37. Cereda E, Klersy C, Rondanelli M, et al. Energy balance in patients with pressure ulcers: a systematic review and meta-analysis of observational studies. J Am Diet Assoc 2011;111(12):1868–76.

38. Lubos Sobotka. Galén. Basics in clinical nutrition. 5th Edition. Galén; 2019. p. 289–91.

39. Kondrup J, Rasmussen HH, Hamberg I, et al. Nutritional risk screening (NRS 2002): a new method based on an analysis of controlled clinical trials. Clin Nutr 2003;3:321–36.

40. Nestle Nutrition Institute. Mini nutritional assessment MNA®. 1994. Available at: www.mna-elderly.com/forms/mini/mna_mini_english.pdf. Accessed September 27, 2021.

41. Hubbard GP, Elia M, Holdoway A, et al. A systematic review of compliance to oral nutritional supplements. Clin Nutr 2012;31(3):293–312.

42. Lobo DN, Gianotti L, Adiamah A, et al. Perioperative nutrition: recommendations from the ESPEN expert group. Clin Nutr 2020;39(11):3211–27.

43. Druml C, Ballmer PE, Druml W, et al. ESPEN guideline on ethical aspects of artificial nutrition and hydration. Clin Nutr 2016;35(3):545–56.

44. O'Sullivan-Maillet J, Schwartz DB, Posthauer ME. Ethical and legal issues in feeding and hydration. J Acad Nutr Diet 2013;113(6):828–33.

The Role of Hyperbaric Oxygen Therapy for the Treatment of Wounds

Merrine Klakeel, DO*, Karen Kowalske, MD

KEYWORDS

- Hyperbaric oxygen therapy • Diabetic wounds • Chronic refractory osteomyelitis
- Radionecrosis

KEY POINTS

- Hyperbaric oxygen therapy (HBOT) is used as an adjunct therapy for the treatment of chronic nonhealing wounds.
- HBOT is a safe and effective therapy when used within the recommended treatment parameters.
- HBOT maximizes the benefits of oxygen and augments the body's natural defense mechanisms to enhance healing.

INTRODUCTION TO HYPERBARIC OXYGEN

Hyperbaric oxygen therapy (HBOT) is used to treat carbon monoxide poisoning, air embolism, decompression sickness, and as an adjuvant treatment for a variety of refractory medical diagnoses including diabetic wounds, osteoradionecrosis, and osteomyelitis[1,2]. For the purposes of this article, we will focus on the benefits of HBO for wound healing.

During HBOT, patients are placed in a pressurized chamber breathing either room air or 100% oxygen while the pressure inside the chamber is increased from 1.4 atm absolute (ATA) to 3 ATA. There are two types of HBO chambers available: multiplace and monoplace. The multiplace chambers allow for multiple patients to dive simultaneously with a staff diver accompanying the dive. In a multiplace environment, the chamber is filled with room air and patients are provided with removable masks to breathe 100% oxygen while the staff is exposed to room air under a pressurized environment. In a monoplace chamber, the patient is placed alone inside the chamber with the whole chamber filled with 100% oxygen (**Fig. 1**).

Department of Physical Medicine and Rehabilitation, UT Southwestern Medical Center, 5151 Harry Hines Boulevard, Dallas, TX, 75390, USA
* Corresponding author.
E-mail address: Merrine.klakeel@utsouthwestern.edu

Phys Med Rehabil Clin N Am 33 (2022) 823–832
https://doi.org/10.1016/j.pmr.2022.06.008
1047-9651/22/© 2022 Elsevier Inc. All rights reserved.

pmr.theclinics.com

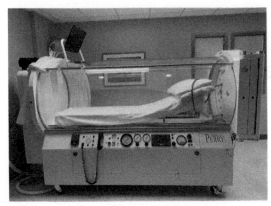

Fig. 1. Monoplace hyperbaric oxygen chamber at UT Southwestern, Medical Center, Dallas, Texas.

To obtain clinical benefit, the chamber pressure must be 1.4 ATA or greater while breathing 100% oxygen.[1] Safe treatments can be ensured for pressures up to 3 ATA for up to 2 h[3,4] at a time to minimize complications such as seizures due to oxygen toxicity. To obtain full benefit of the therapy, the pressurized oxygen must be breathed to allow for saturation of hemoglobin and for oxygen to be dissolved into plasma at high atmospheric pressure. During treatment, the arterial oxygen tension can exceed 2000 mm Hg and tissue oxygen levels can reach up to 200 to 500 mm Hg during HBOT.[3,5] Because the benefit of HBO is derived from oxygen being dissolved into blood plasma at high pressures, topical application of HBO to affected limb superficially does not provide the expected healing and is currently not an approved treatment for Medicare. In general, HBOT protocols involve one to two treatments daily for 1.5 to 2 h at 2 to 2.5 ATA for 20 to 50 days or sessions.[5]

HBO is recommended as primary and adjunct therapies for multiple diagnosis. **Box 1** lists the Medicare-approved diagnosis[6] for HBOT.

Mechanism of Hyperbaric Oxygen Therapy Explained

The molecular details of how HBOT facilitates wound healing through multiple pathways remain to be fully elucidated. To understand how HBOT promotes wound healing, first let's review the mechanisms that promote a nonhealing wound environment. Factors contributing to wound hypoxia in chronic wounds include peripheral vascular disease, increased oxygen demand of healing tissue, and insufficient presence of reactive oxygen species (ROS).[7] Ischemia is the lack of vascular perfusion resulting in hypoxia and loss of nutrient supply.[7] Hypoxia is the reduction of partial pressure of oxygen below tissue demand[7] leading to cell death or chronic state of nonhealing. The hypoxic and ischemic environment provides the ideal condition for bacteria to thrive due to the lack of oxygen-dependent bacterial killing of leukocytes.[8] The increase in tissue oxygen level during HBOT reverses the local tissue injury induced by hypoxia and inflammation.

Increased oxygen promotes the bacterial killing capability of polymorphonuclear leukocytes. Tissue hyperoxia promotes the formation of ROS under oxidative stress and enhances the antimicrobial effects of the immune system.[3,9] ROS are ionized oxygen molecules that are highly reactive. Macrophages and neutrophils use ROS for bacterial killing and phagocytosis.[7,10] ROS such as superoxide anion $.O_2^-$, peroxide $.O_2^{2-}$, hydrogen peroxide H_2O_2, hydroxyl radicals $.OH$, and hydroxyl OH^- ions are

---

Box 1
Approved Medicare diagnosis[6].

1. Acute carbon monoxide intoxication
2. Decompression illness
3. Gas embolism
4. Gas gangrene
5. Acute traumatic peripheral ischemia
6. Crush injuries and suturing of severed limbs
7. Progressive necrotizing infections
8. Acute peripheral arterial insufficiency
9. Preparation and preservation of compromised skin grafts
10. Chronic refractory osteomyelitis, when unresponsive to conventional management
11. Osteoradionecrosis as an adjunct to conventional treatment
12. Soft-tissue radionecrosis as an adjunct to conventional treatment
13. Cyanide poisoning
14. Actinomycosis, as an adjunct to conventional therapy when unresponsive to antibiotics and surgical treatment
15. Diabetic wounds of the lower extremities if all of these apply:
    a. Has Type 1 or Type 2 diabetes and has lower extremity wound associated with diabetes.
    b. Wound classified as Wagner grade III or higher.
    c. Failed adequate course of standard wound therapy.

---

produced by various metabolites within the cell through redox reactions.[3] ROS is antimicrobial by nature and is effective against gram-negative and gram-positive bacteria by inducing damage to cellular DNA, RNA, proteins, and lipid membranes.[3,11] Maximal ROS production occurs intracellularly at tissue oxygen pressure greater than 300 mm Hg, which can only be achieved by breathing supplemental oxygen at higher concentrations than room air.[7]

HBO is bactericidal to anaerobic bacteria because hyperoxia increases the formation of oxygen free radicals, which are lethal to anaerobic metabolisms.[12] HBO displays bacteriostatic effectiveness against aerobic and facultative anaerobic bacteria by impairing the protein synthesis and functions of nucleic acids and membrane transport mechanisms. HBOT assists in modulating infections by heightening the immune system's antimicrobial effects and through additive benefits to antibiotics.[3,9] Kohanski and colleagues[13] showed that although aminoglycosides, quinolones, and β-lactams all have a unique bactericidal mechanism with specific target sites such as ribosomes, DNA gyrase, and glycopeptides, these antibiotics all participate in the tricarboxylic acid (TCA) cycle to generate hydroxyl radicals to promote bactericidal activity. TCA cycle is an aerobic pathway and requires sufficient tissue oxygen levels to function. Tissue hyperoxia affects the activity of antibiotics.[3,8] Turhan and colleagues[12] found that adjunct HBOT to antibiotics vancomycin, teicoplanin, and linezolid in the treatment of MRSA mediastinitis in a rat model increased the effectiveness of each antibiotic significantly compared with the antibiotic alone group.[8] Hyperoxia has been reported to inhibit the growth of some fungi and potentiate the antifungal drug amphthericin B.

Under hyperoxic conditions, cells within wounds increase collagen synthesis, growth factor production, and improve cell migration and tube-formation functions.[5] Angiogenesis requires an extracellular matrix composed of collagen and proteoglycans to guide tube formation and resist the pressure of blood flow. Molecular oxygen is necessary for hydroxylation of proline and lysine to cross-link the collagen necessary for angiogenesis.[7] Hopf and colleagues[14] found that angiogenesis was significantly increased in all hyperoxic groups compared with normoxia groups.

Oxygen as a potent drug potentiates the effects of ATP, downregulates complex molecular cascades involving β-2 integrin and pro-inflammatory cytokines, upregulates anti-inflammatory cytokines and growth factors, and mobilizes stem cells.[15] The increased oxygen from HBOT causes upregulation and downregulation of various growth factors and cytokines such as interferon-γ, interleukin-1(IL-1), IL-6, IL-2, IL-10, and tumor necrosis factor alpha. Fibroblasts promote angiogenesis by producing regulatory factors such as vascular endothelial growth factor (VEGF), stromal cell-derived growth factor-1 (SDF-1), and platelet-derived growth factor (PDGF) that promote proliferation, migration, and tube formation of endothelial cells.[16] In a study by Huang and colleagues fibroblasts treated with 90 min of HBOT for 4 to 5 days showed a higher cell proliferation rate in a diabetic mice model.

HBOT increases the arterial oxygen pressure to 2000 mm Hg and tissue O_2 pressure to 500 mm Hg at 3 ATA.[3,12] HBO induces vasodilation in hypoxic tissues and vasoconstriction in tissue with adequate oxygenation.[15] The increased plasma oxygen is sufficient and arterial vasoconstriction does not induce hypoxia in normal tissue.[17] Hyperoxic vasoconstriction occurs only after severely hypoxic tissues have been corrected, causing elevated blood pressures. Cardiac output and heart rate is reduced to reduce the increase in arterial pressure caused by systemic peripheral vasoconstriction.[12] Anti-edema effects by vasoconstriction decrease leukocyte chemotaxis and adhesion, attenuates ischemia-reperfusion damage, and suppresses the formation of inflammatory mediators that promotes ischemic injury in crush injuries or compartment syndromes.[3,17]

Clinical Application of Hyperbaric Oxygen Therapy in Wound Healing

Diabetic Wounds

Diabetes mellitus and associated foot ulcers are a major cause of impairment and health care expenditure. More than half of these wounds become infected requiring emergency room visits, hospitalization, and potential amputation. Individuals with diabetes who develop a foot ulcer are three times more likely to die in the next year than those without an ulcer.[18] The pathogenesis of diabetic foot ulcers is based on three complications overlapping including neuropathy, angiopathy, and impaired response to infection.[19] The standard of care for these ulcers is to relieve pressure, maximize perfusion, and treat infection, glycemic control, and local wound care. The concept of using HBO for diabetic foot ulcers revolves around the large vessel and small vessel ischemia by increasing tissue oxygen tension and stimulating angiogenesis.[20] A literature review of diabetic foot ulcers and hyperbaric oxygen treatment shows more systematic reviews than actual studies. Also, most of these studies do not have well-defined outcomes. The majority of reviews report on amputation. The two that claim to decrease the rate of amputation are not supported by statistical power.[21]

Despite the inconsistency of prior studies, HBOT is approved by the Center for Medicare and Medicaid Services for the treatment of Wagner 3 diabetic foot ulcers. Careful evaluation of the wounds with adequate supporting diagnoses is essential for avoiding billing denials. The fact that a patient has diabetes must be documented in the medical record and ideally should be listed as a secondary code when billing.

Next, the wound is ideally related to diabetes. This link is relatively easy in a pressure area of the foot in an individual with a diabetic foot ulcer. The physical examination should include peripheral pulses and documentation of sensory changes associated with neuropathy. Understanding the Wagner classification of diabetic foot ulcers is essential. To be a Wagner 3 there must be a deep ulcer with osteomyelitis or abscess. Bone biopsy or deep tissue cultures may be required to meet these criteria. Lastly, conservative treatment must be maximized. Vascular studies showing good perfusion or vascular surgery notes reporting that perfusion is maximized is essential. The infection needs to be addressed and treated. Patients who smoke need to quit before treatment both for wound healing and HBO safety. Documentation of diabetic control should be documented. If hemoglobin A1c is elevated, an appropriate management plan should be recorded. HBOT lowers blood sugar levels acutely so it should always be checked before each dive for someone with diabetes. It is recommended that pre-dive blood sugar should be greater than 120 mg/dL. Patients should reduce or skip morning insulin or oral hypoglycemics to reduce the risk of hypoglycemia during HBOT.[22]

Chronic Refractory Osteomyelitis

Osteomyelitis is an inflammatory process affecting bone due to infiltration of the tissue by bacteria and involves all or some portion of the bone: periosteum, cortical bone, trabecular bone, and bone marrow.[23,24] The Cierny Mader classification system grades osteomyelitis based on the extent of the affected bone. Osteomyelitis can be categorized into three characteristic types based on cause, vascular insufficiency (diabetic foot ulcer), contiguous spread (pressure ulcer or local trauma), and hematogenous spread (vertebral osteomyelitis).[25-27] Acute infection presents within weeks, whereas chronic osteomyelitis persists over months to years.[24] Diagnosis of osteomyelitis is based on the clinical presentation of acute symptoms, fever, chills, malaise, or chronically with recurrent symptoms or nonhealing wounds, often identified on diagnostic imaging workup. Osteomyelitis results from the development of sequestrum, dead bone, and abscess surrounded by avascular bone limiting the penetration of antibiotics and inflammatory cells, rendering them ineffective.[24] Radiographic imaging can detect soft-tissue swelling, bone destruction, and periosteal reaction within 10 to 21 days of infection.[28] MRI can detect bone edema earlier and is more sensitive for the diagnosis of osteomyelitis; however, it cannot be used to track the progress of therapies because of persistent bone edema for months after cure.[28] CT-guided biopsy or surgical bone biopsy provides the best culture sample for minimizing contamination. Swab cultures often grow contaminate and do not correlate with bone biopsy.[24] C-reactive protein can be used to track response to treatment, with the levels dropping to normal within weeks of starting antibiotics.[24]

Owing to the avascular nature of the bone, a lengthy antibiotic course extending weeks to months is necessary for complete treatment. The addition of HBOT as adjunct therapy has been proven to be highly effective in healing osteomyelitis. HBOT uses hyperoxic conditions with increased antimicrobial activity by leukocytes using ROS for bacterial killing while augmenting antibiotics. Treatment of chronic refractory osteomyelitis requires a multidisciplinary team involving a surgical team, infectious disease, and HBO specialist. The tenth European Consensus conference on hyperbaric medicine recommends HBOT for refractory chronic osteomyelitis with Type 1 and level C evidence and likewise for nonhealing wounds related to diabetes and ischemia.[29] Chronic refractory osteomyelitis is an approved diagnosis for HBOT and should be considered as an adjunctive therapy when conventional medical and surgical interventions fail to show improvement in the disease process.

Eltori and colleagues[30] showed a 68% cure rate (30 out of 44 patients) in the treatment of osteomyelitis in spinal cord injury patients with HBOT at 2 ATA for 2 h with 50 average treatments, with follow-up studies from 6 months to 9 years. In a systemic review of literature, Savvidou and colleagues[31] reviewed 20 cohort studies and 20 case studies and found that 308 (73.5%) of the 419 patients who received complete HBOT had a successful outcome without reported relapse. Staphylococcus aureus was the most common pathogen observed in the studies reviewed, but others included Streptococci species, Pseudomonas aeruginosa, Proetus species, Enterococci, Escherichia coli, Staphylococcus epidermidis, Propinoibacterium acnes, Klebsiella species, Serratia species, Clostridia species, and fungi like Candida species, Saccharomyces cerevisiae, and Rhizopus species.[31] Hanley and colleagues[32] recommend a treatment dose of 2.4 ATA for 90 min with 5-min air break every 30 min for 40 to 60 treatment sessions for chronic osteomyelitis (Hanley-HBT chronic RO).

Radionecrosis

Radiation therapy is frequently used for the treatment of cancer along with chemotherapy and surgery. Although radiation therapy targets to destroy malignant cells, adjacent tissue unavoidably absorbs some radiation resulting in acute and chronic injury to the nontargeted soft tissue. Late radiation tissue injury is dose-dependent affecting mostly patients who received greater than 5000 cGy of radiation during treatment and late injury occurs in approximately 5% and 15% of long-term survivors.[33,34]

Acute radiation soft-tissue injury occurs during treatment or within a few weeks of treatment in rapidly proliferating cells such as skin or gastrointestinal tract, when normal cells are destroyed. The acute symptoms include hair loss, erythema, blistering, and ulceration of the skin with symptoms resolving as new cells are replaced by the stem cells.[33,35] Radiation induces ionization of cellular structures and production of free radicals resulting in DNA damage causing cellular death during mitosis.[33,35] Radiation produces proinflammatory cytokines, induces vascular injury, edema, and inflammatory responses and affects wound healing processes leading to chronic tissue changes.[35]

Late or chronic symptoms occur in tissues with slow turnover months to years after radiation therapy and presents with soft-tissue fibrosis, tissue necrosis or atrophy, fistula formation, vascular injury, and impaired wound healing.[34,35] The late effects of radiation are tissue and organ specific.[35] The affected tissue continues to deteriorate with increased fibrosis and loss of vascular supply until the tissue becomes too ischemic to function normally leading to necrosis or skin breakdown. The damage is exacerbated by trauma or infection.[36] Surgery has been considered a definitive treatment; however, it can also lead to a further breakdown, delayed healing, and increased risk of infections.[35,36]

Marx and colleagues[37] showed that HBOT can promote angiogenesis in irradiated tissue when breathing 100% oxygen at 2.4 ATA. Angiogenesis in irradiated tissue is mediated by the migration of macrophages by various biochemical messengers from endothelial cell responses at the injury site. HBOT has shown an 80% response rate with a decrease in fibrosis, stimulates angiogenesis, stimulates stem cells, promotes new granulation tissue growth, reduction in bleeding from ulcerated mucosal tissue, and improved osteocyte functions in radiation-damaged bone.[33,38]

An observational cohort study of the Radionecrosis Research Registry by Niezgoda and colleagues[39] found that osteoradionecrosis, dermal soft-tissue radionecrosis, cystitis, proctitis, and laryngeal radionecrosis were the most common radiation injuries. This study also showed improvement in symptoms by 76.7% to 92.6% post HBOT depending on injury type, with osteoradionecrosis having the highest percent of symptom relief at 92.6% and laryngeal radionecrosis with 76.7% of symptom relief.[39] Bennett and colleagues[36] found moderate-quality evidence that complete mucosal coverage of exposed bone was more likely in osteoradionecrosis with HBOT and that wound dehiscence was less likely following surgical intervention for osteoradionecrosis of the mandible when combined with HBOT. In a review of 67 patient case series with late radiation tissue injury after breast cancer by Spruijt and colleagues,[40] improvements were seen in pain, fibrosis, edema, and shoulder movement scores after HBOT.

Despite the improvement in the quality of tissue overall, it is important to recognize that HBOT cannot restore the tissue to prior normal integrity. Recommended treatment dose for soft-tissue radionecrosis is 30 to 40 treatments at 2 to 3 ATA for 90 to 110 min to promote angiogenesis.[33] Benefit of therapy is seen after about 20 sessions and plateaus at 30 to 40 treatments.[33] Goal of HBOT for Late radiation tissue injury is to reverse ischemia by promoting angiogenesis and improve granulation tissue before pursuing surgical closure or choosing to heal by secondary intention.[33]

Complications of Hyperbaric Oxygen Therapy

HBOT is a safe and effective therapy when used within the recommended treatment parameters. The risks associated with HBOT are associated with hyperoxia and increased pressure during treatment.[17] CNS oxygen toxicity can cause generalized seizures with prolonged exposure to oxygen at pressures higher than 2.8 ATA. Risk of generalized seizure can be reduced by taking room air breaks while inside the chamber. Other complications of HBO include hypertension, hypoglycemia, blurry vision from reversible myopia, and barotrauma to the middle ear, sinuses, teeth, and lungs causing pneumothorax.[12,33,41] Risk of hypoglycemia can be reduced by monitoring blood sugars using diabetic finger sticks before and after dives and adjusting diabetic medications as needed and requesting patients eat before treatment. Barotrauma to the middle ear can be reduced by teaching patients to equalize pressure in their ears during treatment or by referral to Otolaryngologist for tympanostomy tubes. Risk of pulmonary barotrauma can be reduced by confirming the lack of preexisting pneumothorax or blebs using lung imaging studies.[17] Increased chamber pressure can exacerbate congestive heart failure, and obtaining cardiac clearance is justified in patients with poor ejection fraction. Chemotherapeutic agents such as doxorubicin, bleomycin, or cisplatin should be avoided with adjunct HBOT due to interference in mechanisms of free oxygen radicals.[31] History of bleomycin chemotherapy places patients at increased risk of pulmonary fibrosis with HBOT and risk versus benefit must be considered before starting HBOT.[33] Concomitant administration of HBOT and cisplatin is toxic to the bladder and is a contraindication.[33] Malignancy is not a contraindication and HBOT has not been associated with cancer expansion or recurrence.[31] Absolute contraindication includes pneumothorax, restrictive airway disease, and ongoing chemotherapy.[3]

Hyperbaric Oxygen Chamber Certification Requirements

Undersea and hyperbaric medical society (UHMS) offers an accreditation of hyperbaric medicine facilities and is the only hyperbaric-specific accreditation recognized by The Joint Commission. A detailed Accreditation manual is available on the UHMS website. It is a very comprehensive evaluation process. The program evaluates the adequacy of the facility and equipment, the appropriateness of staff and training, quality of care, and safety. Governing regulations, oversite, and finances are also reviewed. Facilities are designated at 3 levels. Level 1 provides emergency care and is open 24 h a week. Level 2 are hospital-affiliated outpatient centers that provide care

5 days per week. Level 3 programs are not hospital affiliated. The Medical Director must be board certified in UHM by ABMS or AOA or have a certificate of added qualifications. All the HBO providers must have completed at least a 40-credit hour UHMS approved hyperbaric medicine introductory course, complete 12 h of Category 1 CME in hyperbaric medicine-related topics each year, and be privileged to practice hyperbaric medicine by the facilities credentialing committee.[42] Facility requirements include meeting standards in facility construction, chamber fabrication and ventilation, fire protection, electrical systems, and gas handling. All hyperbaric personnel must be trained in emergency hyperbaric decompression.

SUMMARY

HBOT maximizes the benefits of oxygen and augments the body's natural defense mechanisms to enhance healing. It is an excellent tool in the toolkit of a wound care physician but should only be used when warranted. To be used appropriately, the provider must understand indications and contraindications, assure that large vessel disease has been appropriately managed, the infection has been treated, and underlying disease management is addressed. Detailed attention to safety issues and documentation are also required to create a successful program.

DISCLOSURES

None.

REFERENCES

1. Moon RE. Hyperbaric oxygen therapy indications. undersea and hyperbaric medical society web site. 2019. Available at: https://www.uhms.org/resources/hbo-indications.html. Accessed May 2, 2021.
2. Benedict Mitnick CD, Johnson-Arbor K. Atypical wounds; hyperbaric oxygen therapy. Clin Podiatr Med Surg 2019;36(3):525–33.
3. Memar MY, Yekani M, Alizadeh N, et al. Hyperbaric oxygen therapy: antimicrobial mechanisms and clinical application for infections. Biomed Pharmacother 2019; 109:440–7.
4. Hunter S, Langemo DK, Anderson J, et al. Hyperbaric oxygen therapy for chronic wounds. Adv Skin Wound Care 2010;23(3):116–9.
5. Thom SR. Hyperbaric oxygen: its mechanisms and efficacy. Plast Reconstr Surg 2011;127(Suppl 1):131s–41s.
6. Medicare.gov. Hyperbaric oxygen therapy. Available at: https://www.medicare.gov/coverage/hyperbaric-oxygen-therapy. Accessed May 2, 2021.
7. Sen CK. Wound healing essentials: let there be oxygen. Wound Repair Regen 2009;17(1):1–18.
8. Turhan V, Sacar S, Uzun G, et al. Hyperbaric oxygen as adjunctive therapy in experimental mediastinitis. J Surg Res 2009;155(1):111–5.
9. Cimşit M, Uzun G, Yildiz S. Hyperbaric oxygen therapy as an anti-infective agent. Expert Rev Anti Infect Ther 2009;7(8):1015–26.
10. Dunnill C, Patton T, Brennan J, et al. Reactive oxygen species (ROS) and wound healing: the functional role of ROS and emerging ROS-modulating technologies for augmentation of the healing process. Int Wound J 2017;14(1):89–96.
11. Dryden M. Reactive oxygen species: a novel antimicrobial. Int J Antimicrob Agents 2018;51(3):299–303.

12. Bitterman H. Bench-to-bedside review: oxygen as a drug. Crit Care 2009; 13(1):205.
13. Kohanski MA, Dwyer DJ, Hayete B, et al. A common mechanism of cellular death induced by bactericidal antibiotics. Cell 2007;130(5):797–810.
14. Hopf HW, Gibson JJ, Angeles AP, et al. Hyperoxia and angiogenesis. Wound Repair Regen 2005;13(6):558–64.
15. Smolle C, Lindenmann J, Kamolz L, et al. The history and development of hyperbaric oxygenation (hbo) in thermal burn injury. Medicina (Kaunas) 2021;57(1).
16. Huang X, Liang P, Jiang B, et al. Hyperbaric oxygen potentiates diabetic wound healing by promoting fibroblast cell proliferation and endothelial cell angiogenesis. Life Sci 2020;259:118246.
17. Gill AL, Bell CN. Hyperbaric oxygen: its uses, mechanisms of action and outcomes. Qjm 2004;97(7):385–95.
18. Saluja S, Anderson SG, Hambleton I, et al. Foot ulceration and its association with mortality in diabetes mellitus: a meta-analysis. Diabet Med 2020;37(2):211–8.
19. Gibbons GW, Shaw PM. Diabetic vascular disease: characteristics of vascular disease unique to the diabetic patient. Semin Vasc Surg 2012;25(2):89–92.
20. Hopf HW, Kelly M, Shapshank D. Oxygen and the basic mechanisms of wound healing. In: Neuman TS, Thom SR, editors. Physiology and medicine of hyperbaric oxygen therapy. 1st edition. Philadelphia, PA: Saunders Elsevier; 2008. p. 25.
21. Vinkel J, Holm NFR, Jakobsen JC, et al. Effects of adding adjunctive hyperbaric oxygen therapy to standard wound care for diabetic foot ulcers: a protocol for a systematic review with meta-analysis and trial sequential analysis. BMJ Open 2020;10(6):e031708.
22. George K, Ross D, Rowe L. Integration of data to establish a standard operating procedure for the diabetic patient undergoing hyperbaric oxygen therapy. J Wound Ostomy Continence Nurs 2017;44(6):546–9.
23. Maffulli N, Papalia R, Zampogna B, et al. The management of osteomyelitis in the adult. Surgeon 2016;14(6):345–60.
24. Lew DP, Waldvogel FA. Osteomyelitis. Lancet 2004;364(9431):369–79.
25. Waldvogel FA, Medoff G, Swartz MN. Osteomyelitis: a review of clinical features, therapeutic considerations and unusual aspects. N Engl J Med 1970;282(4): 198–206.
26. Waldvogel FA, Medoff G, Swartz MN. Osteomyelitis: a review of clinical features, therapeutic considerations and unusual aspects (second of three parts). N Engl J Med 1970;282(5):260–6.
27. Waldvogel FA, Medoff G, Swartz MN. Osteomyelitis: a review of clinical features, therapeutic considerations and unusual aspects. 3. Osteomyelitis associated with vascular insufficiency. N Engl J Med 1970;282(6):316–22.
28. Lam G, Fontaine R, Ross FL, et al. Hyperbaric oxygen therapy: exploring the clinical evidence. Adv Skin Wound Care 2017;30(4):181–90.
29. Mathieu D, Marroni A, Kot J. Tenth european consensus conference on hyperbaric medicine: recommendations for accepted and non-accepted clinical indications and practice of hyperbaric oxygen treatment. Diving Hyperb Med 2017; 47(1):24–32.
30. Eltorai I, Hart GB, Strauss MB. Osteomyelitis in the spinal cord injured: a review and a preliminary report on the use of hyperbaric oxygen therapy. Paraplegia 1984;22(1):17–24.
31. Savvidou OD, Kaspiris A, Bolia IK, et al. Effectiveness of hyperbaric oxygen therapy for the management of chronic osteomyelitis: a systematic review of the literature. Orthopedics 2018;41(4):193–9.

32. Hanley ME, Hendriksen S, Cooper JS. Hyperbaric treatment of chronic refractory osteomyelitis. In: StatPearls. Treasure Island (FL): StatPearls Publishing; 2021. Copyright © 2021, StatPearls Publishing LLC.

33. Buboltz JB, Hendriksen S, Cooper JS. Hyperbaric soft-tissue radionecrosis. In: StatPearls. Treasure Island (FL): StatPearls Publishing; 2021. StatPearls Publishing LLC.; 2021.

34. Borab Z, Mirmanesh MD, Gantz M, et al. Systematic review of hyperbaric oxygen therapy for the treatment of radiation-induced skin necrosis. J Plast Reconstr Aesthet Surg 2017;70(4):529–38.

35. Stone HB, Coleman CN, Anscher MS, et al. Effects of radiation on normal tissue: consequences and mechanisms. Lancet Oncol 2003;4(9):529–36.

36. Bennett MH, Feldmeier J, Hampson NB, et al. Hyperbaric oxygen therapy for late radiation tissue injury. Cochrane Database Syst Rev 2016;4(4):Cd005005.

37. Marx RE, Ehler WJ, Tayapongsak P, et al. Relationship of oxygen dose to angiogenesis induction in irradiated tissue. Am J Surg 1990;160(5):519–24.

38. Feldmeier JJ. Hyperbaric oxygen therapy and delayed radiation injuries (soft-tissue and bony necrosis): 2012 update. Undersea Hyperb Med 2012;39(6):1121–39.

39. Niezgoda JA, Serena TE, Carter MJ. Outcomes of Radiation Injuries Using Hyperbaric Oxygen Therapy: An Observational Cohort Study. Adv Skin Wound Care 2016;29(1):12–9.

40. Spruijt NE, van den Berg R. The effect of hyperbaric oxygen treatment on late radiation tissue injury after breast cancer: a case-series of 67 patients. Diving Hyperb Med 2020;50(3):206–13.

41. Tibbles PM, Edelsberg JS. Hyperbaric-oxygen therapy. N Engl J Med 1996;334(25):1642–8.

42. Society UHM. UHMS hyperbaric facility accreditation program. Available at: https://www.uhms.org/accreditation/accreditation-for-hyperbaric-medicine.html. Accessed October 4, 2021.

A Stepwise Approach to Nonoperative and Operative Management of the Diabetic Foot Ulceration

Katherine M. Raspovic, DPM*, Matthew J. Johnson, DPM, Dane K. Wukich, MD

KEYWORDS

- Diabetic foot ulcer • Total contact cast • Offloading • Surgical offloading
- Achilles tendon lengthening • Charcot neuroarthropathy

KEY POINTS

- Diabetic foot ulceration etiology is often due to multiple factors.
- Initial evaluation should identify underlying etiology and should rule out underlying infection.
- Initial treatment should include debridement, local wound care, and offloading.
- Surgical indications include underlying infection or correction of deformity.

INTRODUCTION

Approximately 15% of people with diabetes mellitus (DM) develop a diabetic foot ulceration (DFU) during their lifetime. Diabetic foot ulcer independently increases a patient's risk for foot infection, hospitalization, and amputation[1] and is negatively associated with self-reported health-related quality of life.[2] The treatment of DFU and the associated complications of infection, hospitalization, and amputation creates a tremendous economic burden on health care systems. According to Rice and colleagues,[3] the added yearly cost for ulcer care was in the range of $9 to 13 billion in the United States in addition to the costs already associated with diabetes.[3] The emotional distress associated with DFU is demonstrated by the fact that patients with diabetes-related foot complications fear amputation more than death.[4]

There are multiple factors that lead to the development of DFU. The ultimate goals of treatment include healing of the ulcer, maintaining or restoring function, improving

Department of Orthopaedic Surgery, UT Southwestern Medical Center, 1801 Inwood Road, Dallas, TX 75309, USA
* Corresponding author.
E-mail address: katherine.raspovic@utsouthwestern.edu

Phys Med Rehabil Clin N Am 33 (2022) 833–844
https://doi.org/10.1016/j.pmr.2022.06.004
1047-9651/22/© 2022 Elsevier Inc. All rights reserved.

pmr.theclinics.com

quality of life, and preventing infection and amputation. It has been estimated that 85% of diabetes-related amputations are preceded by a foot wound. The treatment of patients with DFU is complex and is optimized when a multidisciplinary approach is used. Specialists taking care patients with DFU most often include a wound care physician, foot and ankle surgeon (podiatric or orthopedic), vascular surgery (if needed to optimize circulation), plastic surgery (for soft tissue reconstruction), infectious diseases specialists, wound care nurses, physical/occupational therapists, and pedorthist/orthotists. Each member of this team is necessary to help these patients achieve their best outcome possible when surgical intervention to treat a DFU is necessary.

The goals of this article are to discuss the key aspects of the initial examination, the standard nonoperative treatment, and the operative treatments for patients with DFU.

INITIAL EVALUATION OF THE DIABETIC FOOT ULCERATION

Patient History: Initial evaluation of the DFU begins with a thorough history. The ulcer duration should be documented as well as any potential inciting events such as poor fitting shoes, a change in activity, an injury, or stepping on an object. Oftentimes patients will report that the ulceration appeared after the development of a callus or blister. Prior treatment modalities should be noted and duration of DM, current glycemic control, history of infection, prior hospitalization, and prior surgical interventions. Comorbidities such as renal, cardiac, and peripheral arterial disease (PAD) should be discussed and prior lower extremity vascular interventions such as angioplasty, arterial bypass, or venous ablation procedures. For example, asking the patient about symptoms of claudication may unmask underlying PAD. Most DFUs are painless, and this indicates the presence of sensory neuropathy. Patients should be asked about the type of shoes they typically wear and if they wear diabetic shoes and/or diabetic pressure relieving insoles. When concern for infection is present, systemic complaints such as nausea, vomiting, fever, chills, malaise, or loss of appetite should be documented.

Physical examination: The four key components of the physical examination of the patient with DFU are the skin/dermatological, neurological, vascular, and musculoskeletal examinations. Both feet should be examined for comparison.

Skin/dermatological examination: The dermatological examination begins with identifying and documenting the specific location of the ulceration (ie, distal toes, dorsal/plantar foot, and malleoli). The depth of the DFU should be described including any deep structures that may be exposed (subcutaneous tissue, tendon, muscle, or bone). Whether or not a DFU probes to the level of bone (with a cotton tip applicator or sterile metal probe) is also important to note.[5,6] A "positive probe to bone test" increases the likelihood of osteomyelitis.[5,6] The wound bed should be accurately described (fibrous, granular, and so forth). The amount of granulation tissue or tissue fibrosis should be noted as well as the presence and type of exudate (serous, serosanguinous, and so forth). Inspect for underlying infection by noting presence or absence of the cardinal signs of inflammation (rubor/redness, tumor/swelling, calor/heat, dolor/pain, function laesa/loss of function). Also, note extent of cellulitis if present, the presence of purulent drainage, malodor, or soft tissue emphysema if present. The presence of hyperkeratotic skin/callus formation is a sign of increased pressure to an area. Shear forces can also create DFU. Autonomic neuropathy can also lead to skin changes such as dryness and fissuring. Absent pedal hair growth may be indicative of PAD.

Neurological examination: The 5.07/10g Semmes Weinstein Monofilament is a widely used tool that can be used to detect the presence and extent of peripheral neuropathy.[7] This examination is performed with the patient's eyes closed and they should be asked to say "yes" if they feel the light touch from the monofilament. There are 10 locations on the plantar aspect of each foot that is tested (under the first/second/third toes, under the first/second/third metatarsal heads, two on the plantar arch, the plantar heel and the dorsal foot).[7] Diminished or absent vibratory sensation with a 128-Hz tuning fork at the hallux interphalangeal joint as well as absence of Achilles tendon reflexes are two other ways to evaluate a patient for the presence of peripheral neuropathy.

Vascular examination: The presence or absence of the dorsalis pedis pulse (dorsal aspect of the midfoot just lateral to the tendon of extensor hallucis longus) and the posterior tibial pulse (behind the medial malleolus) should be noted. The capillary refill time should be brisk. The presence or absence of edema should be documented. If pulses are not palpable, a handheld Doppler can be used to evaluate the pedal pulses. Noninvasive arterial studies should be performed if there is any concern for diminished arterial flow (to be discussed in the next section of this article).

Musculoskeletal examination: The musculoskeletal examination is key to identify whether or not a DFUs underlying etiology is due to a musculoskeletal deformity or abnormal biomechanics. A non-plantargrade foot (ie, walking on skin that is not meant to be walked on) is at risk for the development of DFU. The toes should be examined for the presence of contractures such as hammertoes, mallet toes, or claw toes which may be due to motor neuropathy. Any varus or valgus alignment of the foot/ankle should be noted. Muscle strength or the presence of weakness should be noted with dorsiflexion, plantarflexion, inversion, and eversion of the foot/ankle. Tendon contractures should be noted, especially contracture of the Achilles tendon. Achilles tendon contracture may develop in patients with DM due to nonenzymatic glycation resulting in plantar forefoot ulceration (discussed later in this article).[8] The range of motion of the toes, metatarso-phalangeal joints, hindfoot, and ankle should be examined. Collapse of the longitudinal arch with plantar bone prominence is indicative of Charcot neuroarthopathy. The patient should be asked to stand on the ground so that the alignment of the foot/ankle can be assessed. It is helpful to examine both feet to evaluate for any differences.

CLASSIFICATION OF DIABETIC FOOT ULCERATION

DFU classification systems can been developed to not only document the depth of the ulceration but also to help predict prognosis in the setting of infection and PAD. There are several classification systems that are used for DFU. Meggitt–Wagner classification is the original wound classification that classifies depth, infection, and gangrene.[9] The University of Texas classification assesses depth, infection, and ischemia.[9] SINBAD (Site, Ischemia, Neuropathy, Bacterial Infection, Area and Depth) classifies ulceration based on site, ischemia, neuropathy, bacterial infection, and depth.[10] PEDIS (Perfusion, Extent, Depth, Infection, Sensation) describes perfusion, extent, depth, infection, and sensation.[11] The Society of Vascular Surgery developed WiFi (wound, ischemia, infection).[11] A prospective study comparing the University of Texas, SINBAD, Meggitt–Wagner, and the PEDIS scoring systems showed that the classifications had satisfactory inter-rater agreement but the strength of the agreement varied between classifications.[12]

DIABETIC FOOT ULCERATION WORK UP

Radiology/Imaging: Weight-bearing radiographs of the foot and/or ankle should be obtained on initial DFU evaluation to help identify potential structural risk factors of the DFU. One of the major pitfalls is to order non-weight-bearing radiographs, because these do not correlate the site of ulcer with an anatomic abnormality. Potential causes of DFU that can be identified on radiographs include chronic osteomyelitis, a foreign body, bone deformity, or Charcot neuroarthropathy. If there is a concern for osteomyelitis and radiographs are "unremarkable" then advanced imaging should be obtained such as MRI. LaFontaine and colleagues'[13] recent study of 110 patients showed similar diagnostic accuracy between MRI and SPECT/CT (Single-photon emission computed tomography) in diagnosing diabetic foot osteomyelitis (sensitivity and specificity for SPECT/CT were 89% and 35%, respectively; the same values for MRI were 87% and 37%).[13]

Laboratory Testing: If concern for underlying infection is present, the erythrocyte sedimentation rate (ESR) and C-reactive protein (CRP) can provide useful information. In a study by Lavery and colleagues,[14] hospitalized patients with a foot infection who had an ESR of $\geq$60 mm/h (sensitivity of 74%; 95% CI 67–80 and specificity of 56%; 95% CI 48–63) and a CRP level of $\geq$7.9 mg/dL (sensitivity of 49%; 95% CI 41–57 and specificity of 80%; 95% CI 74–86) were likely to have osteomyelitis.[14] It is important to note that the ESR and CRP are sensitive and not specific; therefore, there are other factors/comorbidities such as end-stage renal disease/hemodialysis that can cause elevation of these levels. The complete blood count may detect the presence of leukocytosis. Good glycemic control is necessary for DFU healing and the hemoglobin A1C should be checked. Nutrition should be optimized, and albumin/prealbumin should be checked if there are nutritional concerns.

Vascular Testing: In those with concern for PAD, noninvasive arterial studies detect underlying ischemia. Testing should include the ankle brachial index (ABI), toe brachial index (TBI), and toe pressures.[15] Patients with diabetes may have calcification of the tunica media in lower extremity arteries, resulting in noncompressible vessels and/or falsely elevated measurements. This is particularly prominent in patients with neuropathy and/or renal disease. The smaller arteries of the toes are less impacted by this and therefore the TBI, in addition to the toe pressures, can be more reliable in determining if adequate arterial flow for DFU healing is present. An ABI between 0.9 and 1.4, TBI greater than or equal to 0.70, and great toe pressures greater than 55 mm Hg are considered adequate for healing.[15]

STANDARD NONOPERATIVE TREATMENT OF THE DIABETIC FOOT ULCERATION (NO INFECTION)

Once a DFU has been properly assessed and there are no concerns for infection or PAD, the standard course of treatment includes sharp debridement, local wound care to maintain a healthy wound environment, and offloading.

Debridement: Debridement is performed with sharp instruments such as scalpels, scissors, or curette which removes devitalized tissue, senescent cells, and biofilm to allow for the formation of healthy granulation tissue.[16] This converts a "chronic" wound to an "acute" wound. After thorough debridement, the remaining wound tissue should be red, yellow, and white (granulation tissue/muscle, fat, and tendon/bone, respectively).[16] Steed and colleagues'[17] pivotal study showed that more frequent debridement of DFU was associated with a higher rate of healing.

Dressings: Proper dressings maintain a moist wound environment that is essential for healing, absorbing exudate, and protecting the wound. Patient comfort as well as cost should also be considered. There are a variety of options available for DFU dressings, although the evidence supporting the use of one particular dressing over another is low.[18] The type of dressing used depends on the environment of the DFU (ie, a DFU with increased exudate may require a more absorptive dressing). There are many dressing options such as simple moist gauze, alginates, and antimicrobials to name a few of the many options available for use. The key is to prevent desiccation of the underlying wound bed.

Offloading: Offloading is critical for DFU healing and oftentimes is not well done. *The specific* type of offloading device is most often dependent on the location of the DFU. The total contact cast (TCC) is the "gold standard" offloading device for plantar fore-foot ulceration and works by more evenly distributing pressure to the hindfoot region. The TCC is ideal for offloading because it cannot be removed by the patient. A study by Mueller and colleagues[19] showed significantly higher rates of healing using TCC and Achilles tendon lengthening for the treatment of patients with plantar DFU versus a TTC alone.[19] The TCC can be time-consuming to apply and requires a level of exper-tise for proper application. Armstrong and colleagues[20] described the "instant total contact cast" (0), by wrapping a premade removable cast walker with plaster of Paris to make it nonremovable. The TCC is usually changed weekly because of swelling reduction and loosening. In scenarios where a patient has a DFU that requires more frequent dressing changes (ie, associated with a lot of wound exudate) a removable boot may be more ideal for DFU offloading. DFUs should decrease in size every 4 weeks by roughly 50%.[21] Sheehan and colleagues[21] demonstrated that a DFU is more likely to heal with standard treatment if there is a 50% reduction in surface area by 4 weeks. If the ulceration has not improved in size then it should be reassessed for any potential impediments to healing. Advanced skin substitutes and autogenous grafting can be considered at this time if there are no barriers to healing such as an underlying infection.

Operative Treatment of Diabetic Foot Ulceration

Diabetic foot ulceration and infection: Surgical intervention should be considered for the nonhealing DFU when there is concern for underlying infection or deformity pre-venting healing. As stated earlier, a thorough work up should be completed to evaluate for all potential causes of the DFU, including underlying infection. On clinical examina-tion, an ulceration that probes to the level of bone, the presence of erythema, increased temperature, pain/loss of function, edema, purulence, and malodor are signs of infection. The presence of leukocytosis, elevated erythrocyte sedimentation date, and elevated CRP are key laboratories that should be ordered. In the setting of chronic osteomyelitis, radiographs will show changes to the bone such as cortical disruption. Advanced imaging such as MRI can show changes consistent with osteo-myelitis/abscess when radiographs are normal. The combination of clinical examina-tion findings, abnormal laboratory values, and radiographs/advanced imaging are used in together to diagnose infection.

Surgical intervention for underlying infection: In cases where infection of the bone/soft tissue is present and preventing DFU healing, surgical intervention may be neces-sary to remove nonviable soft tissue and bone to allow for healing. Bone/tissue spec-imens should be obtained during surgery and sent for culture and histopathology to help confirm the presence of infection, identify the bacterial pathogen, and for plan-ning the duration of antibiotic therapy. Oftentimes surgical treatment of infection will require more than one surgical intervention during an inpatient admission to adequately removal all infected and nonviable bone and tissue. The patient may require some level of foot amputation depending on the extent of bone/tissue loss (ie, partial ray amputation, transmetatarsal amputation, Chopart-level amputation). Certain level amputations can lead to foot imbalances due to the loss of a tendon insertion. For example, if the insertion of the peroneus brevis is compromised during a fifth ray amputation (amputation of the fifth toe and a portion or all of the fifth meta-tarsal), over time the foot will develop a varus/supination deformity because the tibialis posterior tendon is no longer opposed. This progressive development of a varus/su-pination deformity can lead to a lateral ulceration. There are several ways to prevent this, such as taking care to leave the insertion site intact (base of the fifth metatarsal) or reimplanting the tendon's insertion to another bone if the fifth metatarsal base must be sacrificed due to infection. Another option is to return to the OR once the infection has been treated and the foot has healed and performs tendon balancing/tendon transfer procedures to prevent the development of deformity in the future. Although tendon balancing/prevention of deformity is important to prevent future ulceration, the primary focus when surgically treating infection is to eradicate all bone/tissue infection first and then manage the resulting imbalances/potential deformity at a later time.

Surgical intervention for foot and ankle deformity correction: Despite standard treat-ment and proper offloading, a percentage of DFUs will not heal due to deformity of the foot and/or ankle. It is important to remember that for every DFU there is a cause. Healing an ulcer without addressing the cause will result in high and unacceptable rates of recurrence. Biomechanical alterations are one of the most common reasons contributing to DFU. There are multiple surgical deformity correction options depend-ing on the location of the deformity.

Digital deformity: Digital contracture deformities develop in patients with DM due to imbalance between the intrinsic and extrinsic musculature of the toes due to the pro-gressive development of peripheral motor neuropathy. These deformities can lead to ulceration at the distal portion of the toes due to overpowering of the flexor tendons or the dorsal aspects of the toes at the proximal interphalangeal joint (PIPJ) and distal interphalangeal joint (DIPJ) due to overpowering of the extensor tendons. The dorsal toe ulcerations are most often caused from pressure from shoe wear. Because of the underlying neuropathy, a patient may not be able to sense whether or not there is too much pressure on their toes from an ill-fitting shoe. If an ulcer is present at the distal plantar toe and the deformity is supple/flexible (ie, no rigid contracture present at the PIPJ or DIPJ; the deformity is manually reducible) then a simple flexor tenotomy can be performed to correct the flexible deformity and take pressure off of the distal toe. This can be done in the office setting or in the operating room. The patient can ambulate after this procedure in a post-op shoe until the small incision on the plantar aspect of the toe is healed (1 to 3 weeks). A retrospective study of 101 feet that under-went flexor tenotomy had a 95% healing rate at an average of 27 days at over 1 year average follow-up.[22] When the digital deformity is rigid/not manually reducible then an arthroplasty or arthrodesis of the affected PIPJ or DIPJ can be performed to correct this. Most often a small wire is used for temporary fixation of the toe and removed at 4 to 6 weeks postoperatively.

Hallux deformity: Deformity of the great toe can also lead to ulceration of the medial eminence of the first metatarsal head as the hallux becomes more laterally deviated over time (hallux valgus). Ulceration can also develop on the plantar aspect of the hallux interphalangeal joint. The Keller arthroplasty (resection of the base of the hallux proximal phalanx) has been used to heal DFU of the medial eminence and plantar hallux. Tamir and colleagues[23] used resection arthroplasty to heal DFU on the plantar aspect of the hallux interphalangeal joint in 20 patients. Average time to healing was 3 weeks.

Achilles tendon lengthening vs gastrocnemius recession: Equinus contracture leads to plantar forefoot ulceration due to increased forces on the plantar forefoot. This may result from either Achilles contracture (both gastrocnemius and soleus contracted) or gastrocnemius contracture alone. Increased plantar forefoot pressure under the metatarsal heads leads to the development of hyperkeratotic skin/callus that subsequently places pressure and shear forces on the underlying healthy tissues, subsequently causing plantar forefoot ulceration to occur. Most often the Achilles tendon is the deforming force in patients with DFU; however, the gastrocnemius alone may be tight rather than the Achilles tendon complex. The Silfverskiöld test[24] (**Fig. 1**) can help determine whether or not the Achilles contracture is causing the equinus deformity of if the equinus deformity is due to a contracted gastrocnemius. The amount of ankle dorsiflexion should be noted with the knee extended and then flexed. If there is an equal amount of dorsiflexion with both extension and flexion of the knee then an Achilles contracture is present. If there is an increased ankle dorsiflexion with the knee flexed (removing the pull of the gastrocnemius), then the gastrocnemius is contracted. An Achilles tendon lengthening is a very powerful procedure that is used to heal plantar forefoot DFU (**Fig. 2**) and can be performed with three small percutaneous incisions (Hoke's triple hemisection). In Mueller and colleagues' study,[19] patients with plantar forefoot ulceration in two treatment groups were studied. One group consisted of patients treated with TCC alone and the other group consisted of patients treated with TCC and Achilles tendon lengthening. Patients in the TCC plus Achilles tendon lengthening group experienced higher rates of plantar forefoot ulcer healing compared with the TCC treatment group as well as lower rates of recurrence. Care must be taken to ensure that the Achilles tendon is not overlengthened when performing this procedure. If the tendon is overlengthened or ruptures, a "calcaneal gait" can result, leading to increased pressure on the calcaneus when ambulating (**Fig. 3**). This can lead to the development of a plantar heel ulceration which can be difficult to treat.

Charcot foot deformity: Charcot neuroarthropathy was originally described by Jean-Martin Charcot in the 1800s in patients with neuropathy due to tertiary syphilis (**Fig. 4**).[25] It is a condition of the neuropathic foot and/or ankle where a patient

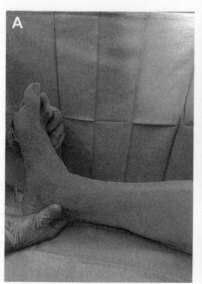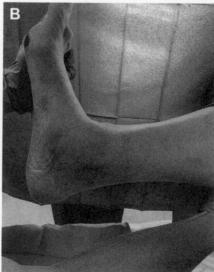

Fig. 1. Performing the Silfverskiold test. (*A*) Ankle in dorsiflexion with knee extended. (*B*) Ankle in dorsiflexion with knee flexed; there is the same amount of dorsiflexion with the knee extended and flexed; therefore, this patient underwent Achilles tendon lengthening for treatment of their non-plantar forefoot ulceration.

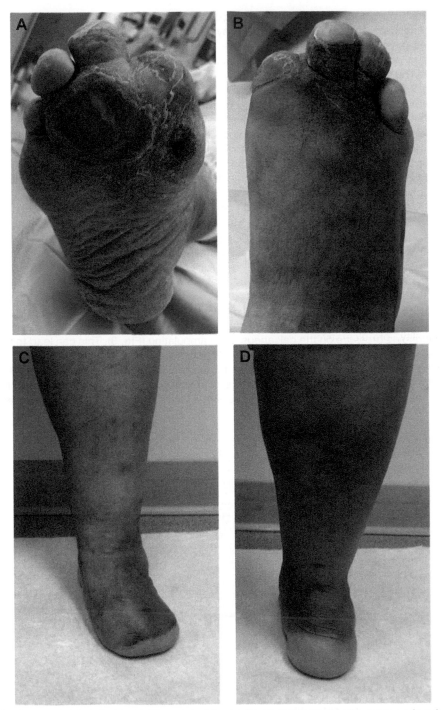

Fig. 2. Dorsal (*A*) and plantar (*B*) aspect of foot with chronic plantar ulceration and underlying osteomyelitis. Patient underwent staged transmetatarsal amputation to treat underlying osteomyelitis followed by Achilles tendon lengthening to decrease forefoot pressure. Patient healed; clinical photos from the front and back (*C, D*).

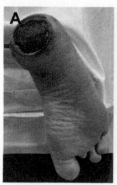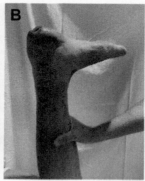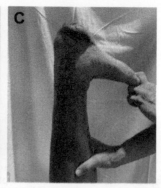

Fig. 3. (A) Patient with plantar calcaneal ulceration due to calcaneal gait that developed as a result of an Achilles tendon rupture that occurred after an Achilles tendon lengthening procedure. Achilles tendon lengthening was originally performed to heal a plantar forefoot ulceration (B) and (C). Note the increase in plantarflexion in figure (C) compared with figure (B).

experiences a known or in many causes unknown or even subtle injury to the foot/ ankle that results in an inflammatory response. This inflammatory response can then progress to osseous weakness, bone/joint collapse, and severe deformity. General indications for surgery in the patient with Charcot include worsening of deformity, instability, pre-ulcerative lesion/impending ulceration, nonhealing, ulceration, and infection. The goals of surgery are to treat infection of present, heal an ulcer if present, and correct the deformity to achieve a plantigrade foot/ankle that can be braced. The ultimate goal of the intervention is to prevent amputation and improve patient quality of life. Patients with Charcot and ulceration have a 12 times greater risk for amputation compared with patients without ulceration.[26] Plantar midfoot ulceration can develop in the setting of midfoot Charcot neuroarthropathy due to the deformity, and these ulcerations may not heal with standard care/offloading. An exostectomy of the prominent plantar bone via a direct approach (excision of the DFU and then removal of the exostosis through this incision) or an indirect approach (separate incision away from the ulceration) is a surgical option to remove the source of pressure and allow for healing.[27] Catanzariti and colleagues [27] showed the decreased recurrence of DFU with removal of a plantar medial exostosis compared with a plantar lateral exostosis.[27] Another option to correct deformity resulting from midfoot Charcot neuroarthropathy that is preventing healing of a plantar midfoot ulceration is realignment arthrodesis. Ankle/hindfoot Charcot deformity can lead to ulceration on the medial/ lateral malleoli. Ankle/hindfoot Charcot deformities are often unstable and are not often amenable to bracing/offloading, leading to more prompt surgical intervention. In general, when there is no concern for infection/proper work up has been performed then internal fixation can be used for surgical reconstruction deformities that are the result of Charcot neuroarthropathy.[28] If there is concern for infection then an external fixation device is used for surgical correction/fixation.

AFTER THE DIABETIC FOOT ULCERATION HEALS

Once the DFU has healed, whether or not they have had surgical intervention to heal, the lower extremity must be protected to prevent re-ulceration or new ulcer development. Depending on the foot type/clinical scenario, some patients only require a diabetic accommodative orthotic and extra-depth shoes. If a patient has residual

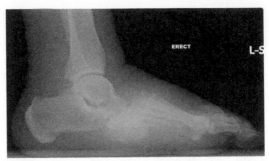

Fig. 4. Patient with midfoot Charcot neuroarthropathy and deformity of the midfoot/collapse of the cuboid leading to plantar lateral ulceration.

deformity or they have had extensive osseous reconstruction (ie, Charcot reconstruction) they may require long-term or life custom shoes, bracing in the form of an ankle-foot orthosis, double upright bracing, or Charcot Restraint Orthotic Walker. Patient should also be closely monitored by a foot and ankle surgeon/specialist after the DFU is healed so that any recurrence or new concern can be promptly identified.

SUMMARY

Treatment of the DFU is complex and multifactorial; however, healing rates are high if the providers appropriately debride the wound, off-load the wound, and create an optimal wound environment for healing. Unfortunately, recurrence is high especially if the underlying etiology is not addressed. The initial evaluation is critical to determine the underlying causes for the DFU and to determine whether or not infection is present. Standard treatment includes sharp debridement, offloading, and maintaining a healthy environment that promotes healing, and a 50% reduction in wound size is expected within 4 weeks. If the wound does not reduce by 50%, reassessment and alternative strategies are necessary. DFU resulting from deformity generally requires surgical correction of the deformity for healing to occur and to reduce the rate of recurrence. The type of surgery depends on the location of the DFU as well as the presence or absence of underlying infection. The goal when treating the patient with DFU is to heal the ulceration, prevent amputation, and return the patient to premorbid function.

CLINICS CARE POINTS

- Treatment of the DFU is complex and multifactorial.
- Initial evaluation is critical to determine the underlying causes for the DFU and to determine whether or not infection is present.
- Standard treatment includes sharp debridement, offloading, and maintaining a healthy environment that promotes healing, and a 50% reduction in wound size is expected within 4 weeks.
- If the wound does not reduce by 50%, reassessment and alternative strategies are necessary.
- DFU resulting from deformity generally requires surgical correction of the deformity for healing to occur and to reduce the rate of recurrence. The type of surgery depends on the location of the DFU as well as the presence or absence of underlying infection.

DISCLOSURE

D.K. Wukich is a consultant for Orthofix, Stryker Wright and receives royalties from Arthrex. He is also on the executive board of the International Association of Diabetic Foot Surgeons. K.M. Raspovic is a consultant for Orthofix. M.J. Johnson has no disclosures.

REFERENCES

1. Lavery LA, Armstrong DG, Wunderlich RP, et al. Risk factors for foot infections in individuals with diabetes. Diabetes Care 2006;29(6):1288–93.
2. Raspovic KM, Hobizal KB, Rosario BL, et al. Midfoot charcot neuroarthropathy in patients with diabetes: the impact of foot ulceration on self-reported quality of life. Foot Ankle Spec 2015;8(4):255–9.
3. Rice JB, Desai U, Cummings AK, et al. Burden of diabetic foot ulcers for medicare and private insurers. Diabetes Care 2014;37(3):651–8.
4. Wukich DK, Raspovic KM, Suder NC. Patients with diabetic foot disease fear major lower-extremity amputation more than death. Foot Ankle Spec 2018;11(1): 17–21.
5. Lavery LA, Armstrong DG, Peters EJ, et al. Probe-to-bone test for diagnosing diabetic foot osteomyelitis: reliable or relic? Diabetes Care 2007;30(2):270–4.
6. Grayson ML, Gibbons GW, Balogh K, et al. Probing to bone in infected pedal ulcers. A clinical sign of underlying osteomyelitis in diabetic patients. JAMA 1995; 273(9):721–3.
7. Armstrong DG, Lavery LA, Vela SA, et al. Choosing a practical screening instrument to identify patients at risk for diabetic foot ulceration. Arch Intern Med 1998; 158(3):289–92.
8. Grant WP, Sullivan R, Sonenshine DE, et al. Electron microscopic investigation of the effects of diabetes mellitus on the Achilles tendon. J Foot Ankle Surg 1997; 36(4):272–8 [discussion: 330].
9. Oyibo SO, Jude EB, Tarawneh I, et al. A comparison of two diabetic foot ulcer classification systems: the Wagner and the University of Texas wound classification systems. Diabetes Care 2001;24(1):84–8.
10. Leese GP, Soto-Pedre E, Schofield C. Independent observational analysis of ulcer outcomes for SINBAD and university of texas ulcer scoring systems. Diabetes Care 2021;44(2):326–31.
11. Bravo-Molina A, Linares-Palomino JP, Vera-Arroyo B, et al. Inter-observer agreement of the Wagner, University of Texas and PEDIS classification systems for the diabetic foot syndrome. Foot Ankle Surg 2018;24(1):60–4.
12. Camilleri A, Gatt A, Formosa C. Inter-rater reliability of four validated diabetic foot ulcer classification systems. J Tissue Viability 2020;29(4):284–90.
13. La Fontaine J, Bhavan K, Lam K, et al. Comparison Between Tc-99m WBC SPECT/CT and MRI for the Diagnosis of Biopsy-proven Diabetic Foot Osteomyelitis. Wounds 2016;28(8):271–8.
14. Lavery LA, Ahn J, Ryan EC, et al. What are the optimal cutoff values for ESR and CRP to diagnose osteomyelitis in patients with diabetes-related foot infections? Clin Orthop Relat Res 2019;477(7):1594–602.
15. Wukich DK, Shen W, Raspovic KM, et al. Noninvasive arterial testing in patients with diabetes: a guide for foot and ankle surgeons. Foot Ankle Int 2015;36(12): 1391–9.
16. Endara M, Attinger C. Using color to guide debridement. Adv Skin Wound Care 2012;25(12):549–55.

17. Steed DL, Donohoe D, Webster MW, et al. Effect of extensive debridement and treatment on the healing of diabetic foot ulcers. Diabetic ulcer study Group. J Am Coll Surg 1996;183(1):61–4.

18. Vas P, Rayman G, Dhatariya K, et al. Effectiveness of interventions to enhance healing of chronic foot ulcers in diabetes: a systematic review. Diabetes Metab Res Rev 2020;36(Suppl 1):e3284.

19. Mueller MJ, Sinacore DR, Hastings MK, et al. Effect of Achilles tendon lengthening on neuropathic plantar ulcers. A randomized clinical trial. J Bone Joint Surg Am 2003;85(8):1436–45.

20. Armstrong DG, Short B, Espensen EH, et al. Technique for fabrication of an "instant total-contact cast" for treatment of neuropathic diabetic foot ulcers. J Am Podiatr Med Assoc 2002;92(7):405–8.

21. Sheehan P, Jones P, Giurini JM, et al. Percent change in wound area of diabetic foot ulcers over a 4-week period is a robust predictor of complete healing in a 12-week prospective trial. Plast Reconstr Surg 2006;117(7 Suppl):239S–44S.

22. Schmitz P, Scheffer R, De Gier S, et al. The Effect of Percutaneous Flexor Tenotomy on Healing and Prevention of Foot Ulcers in Patients With Claw Deformity of the Toe. J Foot Ankle Surg 2019;58(6):1134–7.

23. Tamir E, Tamir J, Beer Y, et al. Resection Arthroplasty for Resistant Ulcers Underlying the Hallux in Insensate Diabetics. Foot Ankle Int 2015;36(8):969–75.

24. Singh D. Nils Silfverskiold (1888-1957) and gastrocnemius contracture. Foot Ankle Surg 2013;19(2):135–8.

25. Sanders LJ. The Charcot foot: historical perspective 1827-2003. Diabetes Metab Res Rev 2004;20(Suppl 1):S4–8.

26. Sohn MW, Stuck RM, Pinzur M, et al. Lower-extremity amputation risk after charcot arthropathy and diabetic foot ulcer. Diabetes Care 2010;33(1):98–100.

27. Catanzariti AR, Mendicino R, Haverstock B. Ostectomy for diabetic neuroarthropathy involving the midfoot. J Foot Ankle Surg 2000;39(5):291–300.

28. Vasukutty N, Jawalkar H, Anugraha A, et al. Correction of ankle and hind foot deformity in Charcot neuroarthropathy using a retrograde hind foot nail-The Kings' Experience. Foot Ankle Surg 2018;24(5):406–10.

Shoe and Bracing Considerations for the Insensate Foot
Shoe considerations for diabetic foot

Daniel Moon, MD, MS[a],*, Ning Cao, MD[b,1], Bianca Martinez, MD[c,1]

KEYWORDS

- Diabetic neuropathy • Prevention of diabetic foot ulcers • Shoe modifications

KEY POINTS

- The development of diabetic foot ulcers is associated with long-term complications of diabetes mellitus, including peripheral neuropathy, peripheral vascular disease, and consequential musculoskeletal and gait abnormalities.
- The goal of therapeutic shoe modifications in diabetic neuropathy is to decrease the amount of time spent on the forefoot during the stance phase and increase total plantar surface area in contact with the ground to distribute pressure appropriately. Three key modifications include extra-depth footwear, metatarsal modifications, and rocker bottom soles.
- Suitably designed and customized footwear has been proven to reduce forefoot plantar pressures and risk of re-ulceration.
- The greatest challenge in creating appropriate shoe modifications is in evaluating the actual forces that lead to tissue breakdown to accurately place the modifications for the optimal decrease in plantar pressures.

EPIDEMIOLOGY OF DIABETIC FOOT COMPLICATIONS

The American Diabetes Association estimates that more than 60,000 lower extremity amputations are performed yearly on the 16 to 18 million individuals with diabetes in the United States. Eighty-five percent of diabetes-associated amputations are preceded by the development of foot ulcers. Fifteen percent of diabetic individuals will develop a foot ulcer or foot infection at some point in their life.[1,2] The primary risk factor for the development of a diabetic foot ulcer is peripheral neuropathy. Other risk

[a] Sheer Gait and Motion Analysis Laboratory and Motor Control Analysis Laboratory, MossRehab, 60 Township Line Road, Elkins Park, PA 19027, USA; [b] MossRehab, Elkins Park, PA, USA; [c] Temple/MossRehab Department of Physical Medicine and Rehabilitation, Philadelphia, PA, USA
[1] Present address: 60 Township Line Road, Elkins Park 19027.
* Corresponding author. 60 Township Line Road, Elkins Park 19027.
E-mail address: Daniel.moon@jefferson.edu

Phys Med Rehabil Clin N Am 33 (2022) 845–856
https://doi.org/10.1016/j.pmr.2022.06.012
1047-9651/22/© 2022 Elsevier Inc. All rights reserved.

factors include peripheral vascular disease, history of the previous amputation, and bony/mechanical deformities (ie, hammertoes and bony prominences).[3–5] To decrease the risk for the development of diabetic foot ulcers and lower extremity amputations, preventative strategies should be used such as patient education, skin and nail care, and therapeutic footwear. The goal of this article was to review the pathophysiology responsible for the development of diabetic foot ulcers and how we can use this knowledge to create protective footwear to prevent the development and recurrence of diabetic foot ulcers.

NORMAL ADULT FOOT ANATOMY AND FUNCTION

A normal gait cycle requires a complex coordination of joint motion and stability, load transfers, and motor control, all of which vary throughout the gait cycle. Diabetic patients with peripheral neuropathy may develop numerous foot deformities that alter the normal gait cycle and cause abnormal distribution of plantar pressures in the foot, thereby predisposing them to diabetic foot ulcers.

The foot is composed of 26 bones and can be divided into the hindfoot, midfoot, and forefoot. The hindfoot includes the tibiotalar joint that is responsible for dorsiflexion and plantarflexion, and the talocalcaneal joint (subtalar joint) that is responsible for inversion and eversion. The midfoot includes the transverse tarsal joint (Chopart joint), and the naviculocuneiform joint and is the location of the center of gravity during normal standing. The forefoot includes the tarsometatarsal joint (Lisfranc joint) and the metatarsal phalangeal joints. The foot has three notable arches: the medial longitudinal, the lateral longitudinal, and the transverse arch. The ligaments (ie, Spring ligament, long and short plantar ligaments) and plantar fascia function as tie beams in maintaining these arches. The foot serves as a sensory interface with the environment. It also has fat pads that help absorb and distribute the shock during weight-bearing.

During the normal gait cycle, the foot facilitates forward propulsion and stability by alternating between a rigid and flexible conformation through the Windlass mechanism and subtalar joint inversion and eversion.[6] The flexible foot conformation allows binding to uneven surfaces for balance and provides shock absorption. When the heel strikes the ground to initiate stance phase, the ankle is pronated, which is characterized by subtalar eversion, ankle dorsiflexion, and forefoot abduction. This creates a preloading effect on the plantar aponeurosis during the transition to the midstance phase. During midstance, the tension in the plantar aponeurosis reduces and the foot can more readily absorb shock and adapt to the terrain through midfoot supination or pronation. During the latter part of the stance phase, the Windlass mechanism occurs which consists of extension of the hallux leading to tightening of the plantar aponeurosis and increased stiffness of the foot. In a terminal stance, the foot is supinated and mechanically locked. This allows the quadriceps muscle to extend the knee against a rigid foot during the transition to push-off or terminal stance phase more efficiently.[6,7]

PATHOPHYSIOLOGY OF DIABETIC FOOT ULCERS

The development of diabetic foot ulcers is multifactorial and associated with long-term complications of diabetes mellitus, including peripheral neuropathy, peripheral vascular disease, and consequential musculoskeletal and gait abnormalities.[8,9]

Among people in the United States older than 40 years of age, peripheral vascular disease is more than twice as prevalent in people with diabetes (10%) than without (.5%).[10] Decreased blood flow lowers tissue oxygenation and impedes proper wound healing, which can contribute to ulceration. Diabetes also causes peripheral neuropathy, affecting sensory, motor, and autonomic nerves. Peripheral sensory neuropathy can lead to the loss of light touch feeling, vibration perception, and protective sensation including pain. A lack of protective sensation can be measured by insensitivity to the Semmes-Weinstein 5.07 (10 g) monofilament.[11] In the absence of protective sensation, trauma to the foot may occur without the patient noticing. Peripheral motor neuropathy can affect both the intrinsic and extrinsic muscles of the lower extremity. The smaller motor nerves in the foot are affected first.[12] The ankle and toe dorsiflexor muscles are smaller and are therefore affected earlier in the disease process than the plantarflexor muscles. This imbalance between the dorsiflexors and plantarflexors results in a dynamic ankle plantarflexed posture during the stance phase, thereby increasing the plantar pressures at the forefoot. Pressure becomes concentrated under the heads of the metatarsals, which contributes to the development of foot ulcers at these sites. Motor nerves are also responsible for the smooth muscle tone of the blood vessels. Thus, if they are damaged there is diminished tone leading to less return of venous fluid which causes soft tissue swelling and if there is also arteriovenous shunting, elevated temperature, erythema, and dilated dorsal veins. The increased blood flow in turn causes monocyte and osteoclast enrichment leading to increased bone resorption, osteopenia, and local bony destruction.[13] In addition, autonomic neuropathy can lead to loss of sweating in the foot which causes dry, cracked feet placing the patient at increased risk for the development of pressure injuries, wounds, and infections.

MUSCULOSKELETAL ABNORMALITIES

Longstanding peripheral neuropathy and peripheral vascular disease associated with diabetes mellitus can lead to the development of several musculoskeletal abnormalities that further increase the risk of diabetic foot ulcers due to aberrant loading. One of the most common foot deformities associated with diabetes mellitus are the hammer and claw toe deformities.[14,15] Studies have shown that subjects with hammer and claw toes have elevated plantar pressures and thinner plantar soft tissue beneath the metatarsal heads but thicker soft tissue beneath the phalanges which displaces the fat pad distally, all of which predispose the patient to develop ulcers under the metatarsal heads.[16]

Other foot structure deformities associated with diabetic foot ulcers include compensated forefoot varus (with subtalar joint pronation), uncompensated forefoot varus, forefoot valgus, and the Charcot foot. Charcot foot, also known as Charcot neuropathic osteoarthropathy, is a rare complication of neuropathy that can lead to the collapse of the arch and rocker bottom foot deformity. In a study correlating ulcer location and foot deformities, patients with plantar ulcers were divided into the following groups: Charcot foot, compensated forefoot varus, uncompensated forefoot varus, or forefoot valgus. This study found that Charcot feet were more likely to have mid-foot ulcers. Feet with compensated forefoot varus tended to have ulcers under the second, third, or fourth metatarsal heads, whereas feet with uncompensated forefoot varus or forefoot valgus had ulcers under the fifth or first metatarsal heads, respectively.[17]

The Achilles tendon and plantar fascia are also frequently found to be abnormally thick in diabetic patients with neuropathy which contributes to the rigid confirmation of the foot leading to poor shock absorption during landing.[18,19] A study examining structural alterations of the main tendinous and ligamentous structures of the foot-ankle complex in the presence of mild-to-severe diabetic neuropathy found that the thicker the Achilles tendon and plantar fascia become, the more the first metatarsophalangeal joint mobility is reduced resulting in more severe alterations in foot loading during gait. More specifically, concurrent changes of the above factors accounted for 70.1% of the changes in loading at the metatarsal heads for all diabetic groups, with and without neuropathy. The foot-loading alterations may be well explained by the earlier onset of the Windlass mechanism in stance phase resulting in a more rigid foot. These patients may also develop a foot slap or uncontrolled rapid plantarflexion following heel strike due to weak ankle dorsiflexors and tight Achilles' tendon. As a major consequence, the loading pattern shows a peculiar early loading of the metatarsal heads shortly after heel strike and a prolonged loading during propulsion. This issue is compounded as the foot structure becomes rigid and transmits high stresses, both compressive and tangential, to the plantar soft tissue.[20]

One of the most severe musculoskeletal complications of neuropathy is Charcot foot. It most commonly affects the foot and is due to the interaction of neuropathy, osteopenia, and proinflammatory cytokines on a calcified peripheral vasculature that maintains its ability to vasodilate despite widespread arteriosclerosis. This arthropathy is most likely triggered by unrecalled trauma that triggers an inflammatory cascade in about two-thirds of affected patients.[21] Trauma can cause microfractures, subluxations, or dislocations, which causes abnormal joint loading and further joint damage that if left untreated can lead to collapse of the arch and rocker bottom foot deformity. The diagnosis of Charcot neuroarthropathy is essentially clinical given the nonspecificity of radiological and biochemical findings in the acute stages. Sanders and Frykberg introduced the anatomical classification of the Charcot foot. In stage 1, the metatarsophalangeal joints are affected; in stage 2, the Lisfranc joint is affected; in stage 3, the Chopart joint is affected; in stage 4, the ankle and the subtalar joint are affected; and the calcaneus is included in stage 5.[22] Early identification and treatment is key to preventing a Chopart foot from progressing.

THE EFFECT OF DIABETES ON THE KINEMATICS AND KINETICS OF GAIT

Several studies have shown that changes in sensory perception due to peripheral neuropathy can cause changes in gait patterns.[23] Patients with diabetic neuropathy have a slower gait, reduced cadence and step length, decreased peak accelerations, a decreased push-off vertical force, and a less rhythmic gait pattern.[24] All these characteristics indicate an apropulsive or "cautious" walking pattern. In addition, diabetic individuals also have limited joint mobility at the tibiotalar, subtalar joint, and the first metatarsophalangeal joint, contributing to gait abnormalities and increased plantar pressures.[25] A study examined the foot-to-floor interaction during gait in terms of center of pressure (COP) to identify the abnormal gait characteristics of diabetic patients with and without peripheral neuropathy. The spatial evolution of COP along the longitudinal axis of the foot was found to be influenced by the articular mobility of tibiotalar and metatarsophalangeal joints in the sagittal plane. The COP spatial evolution in neuropathic patients demonstrated a significantly reduced excursion both longitudinally and mediolaterally. However, healthy subjects showed a COP progression that starts from the heel, passes through the metatarsals, reaches the anterior and medial part of the foot, and ends in the hallux. Diabetic patients with severe neuropathy approach the floor with the most anterior part of the heel and perform push-off at the metatarsals, as shown by the reduction of the COP progression along the longitudinal axis. The resulting gait is like a flat-footed gait, which is characterized by a minimal heel strike and push-off. The neuropathic group also showed a significant reduction of the COP trajectory along the mediolateral axis and a concurrent shift of the loading pattern from the lateral toward the medial part of the foot. This premature load shift toward the medial part of the foot creates a feeling of instability at the ankle that causes a greater stiffness mainly in the frontal plane. These findings support the hypothesis of a substantial change in the functionality of the whole ankle complex, causing a functional flat foot and the acquisition of a hip-based walking strategy in patients with diabetic neuropathy.

Allet et al. studied the gait of diabetic patients in a challenging natural environment with the use of body-worn sensors. When comparing diabetic patients with peripheral neuropathy to healthy controls, all parameters of gait studied (velocity, cadence, stance, double support time, gait cycle time, and stride) were significantly different except for shank and knee angle. No differences in gait parameters were observed between diabetic patients with peripheral neuropathy and those without.[24]

PREVENTION OF DIABETIC FOOT ULCERS

Prevention of diabetic foot ulcers requires foot-specific patient education, prophylactic professional skin, and nail care usually with regular podiatric follow-up, and the use of appropriate protective footwear in addition to medical management of hyperglycemia itself.

BEHAVIORAL MODIFICATIONS

An important aspect of preventing diabetic foot ulcers is patient education. It is imperative to counsel the diabetic patient on smoking cessation and adequate glycemic control to prevent peripheral vascular disease and peripheral neuropathy which contribute to the development of diabetic foot ulcers. It is recommended to perform an annual screen for loss of protective sensation using the Semmes-Weinstein monofilament test. A study compared three walking patterns that can be used to reduce the forefoot peak plantar pressures. A shuffling gait pattern can decrease the peak plantar pressures under the first and second metatarsals (up to 57.8%) and the hallux (up to 63.2%). A hip pull-off pattern can decrease the peak plantar pressures at the forefoot (up to 27%), and a step-to walking pattern can decrease the peak plantar pressures at the forefoot (up to 53%). These walking patterns may be useful to help prevent or heal forefoot ulcers in people with diabetic neuropathies who are most at risk for skin breakdown. Alteration of the walking pattern should be considered for reducing forefoot peak plantar pressures in people with diabetic neuropathies who continue to have ulcers despite protective footwear or in people who are unable or unwilling to wear appropriate footwear and have newly healed plantar ulcers.[26] Another study demonstrated that a slower walking velocity was associated with lower plantar pressures as the vertical ground reaction force increased with faster walking velocities.[27] Thus, another approach for certain patients would be to ask that they walk slower.

DIABETIC FOOTWEAR

The goal of therapeutic shoe modifications in diabetic neuropathy is to decrease the amount of time spent on the forefoot during the stance phase and increase the total plantar surface area in contact with the ground to distribute shock appropriately. A study of 400 diabetic patients with a history of healed ulceration showed that 50% of women and 27% of men wore shoes classified as dangerous (shallow or narrow toe box, no laces, open toes or heels, or heel height placing undue pressure on the ball of the foot) at some point during the day.[28] As previously discussed, increased plantar pressures during locomotion contribute to the development of diabetic foot ulcers. This is compounded by forefoot structural deformities that are prevalent in diabetics that can further increase in-shoe plantar pressures at the metatarsal heads. Guidelines recommend that people with diabetes wear appropriate "diabetic footwear" designed to reduce repetitive stresses that lead to diabetic foot ulcers.[29] However, the guidelines do not identify the best insole design or feature and footwear specification or modification to reduce plantar pressures for foot ulcer prevention in people with diabetes and neuropathy. A systematic review and meta-analyses of 54 studies identified the best footwear and insole design features for offloading the plantar surface of the foot to prevent foot ulceration in people with diabetic peripheral neuropathy.[30] More specifically, the review identified key design features of footwear and insoles regarding profile and shape, material type and properties, modifications, and fabrication techniques, which are discussed below. Heterogeneity was found among the profile, modifications, material, and fabrication techniques used in insoles and footwear design. The studies highlighted the lack of a systematic approach to combining these features, which makes it difficult to distinguish the effectiveness of individual features in offloading plantar foot pressures. There were variations in outcome measures, study design, and quality, making meaningful comparison difficult.

Profile/Shape of the Insole

It is important to increase the softness and cushioning of the insole to evenly distribute plantar pressures, which supplements the function of the fat pads that can atrophy with age and neuropathy. By conforming to the shape of the foot, this allows a reduction in pressure by increasing the area over which the force is applied. It will also dampen the impact of the foot on the ground which leads to decreased forces. To decrease friction and thus shear forces, the outsole should never be more flexible than the foot. A rigid outsole or shank can reduce MTP and TMT dorsiflexion in the stance phase and thereby reduce pressure concentration under the metatarsal heads. Regarding the profile and shape of the insole, two types of profile features were described in the review–an arch and a rocker. The use of an arch profile replicating the contour of the plantar surface of the foot has traditionally been the "gold standard" for insole design for reducing pressure in the diabetic neuropathic foot. The review found that 98% of studies reported using an arch profile as part of the insole configuration, although inconsistency exists in the reporting of the specifications. The meta-analysis provides evidence that an arch profile when added to an insole can enhance the offloading effect by a further 37 kPa when compared with an insole without an arch profile. It is postulated that increasing contact with the plantar surface of the foot allows increased distribution of force over a greater area of the foot, thus plantar foot pressure is reduced.[31]

Rocker bottom outsoles were also commonly studied in these studies. A rocker bottom sole functions to "rock" the foot from heel to toe without bending the shoe. This restores some of the ankle and foot motion that is lost through deformity or stiffness. It also decreases the sagittal motion of the MTP joint and decreases the pressure on the metatarsal heads. There are a variety of rocker-bottom soles that are used to prevent diabetic foot complications. Many of these studies modified the rocker profile of the shoe as a method of reducing peak pressure, particularly under the metatarsal heads. Some success was also achieved in reducing pressure under the second to fourth MTPJ with a negative toe rocker with the apex set at 50%–60% of total shoe length. This resulted in alterations to the forefoot loading pattern, specifically reducing pressure under the metatarsal heads by 30%- 50%.[32,33] The use of a rocker bottom sole could be beneficial in reducing peak pressure in the diabetic neuropathic foot.

However, since pressures in some regions can also be elevated by this type of footwear, attention to individual design for each patient is critical.

Fabrication Techniques Used for the Insole and Shoe

Two different fabrication techniques for insoles and footwear were identified in the review, casting and kinetic informed. Casting is traditionally used to capture the geometric shape of the patient's' foot to 'customize' the insole. At the time, only one study examined the role of three types of casting technique in reducing peak pressure. The authors reported an insole formed from a semi-weight-bearing foot shape offered the greatest peak pressure reduction compared with full-weight-bearing and non-weight-bearing foot shapes, although this difference was not statistically significant.[31] However the remaining studies using a casting approach were not able to find any improvement in reducing pressure using the semi-weight-bearing foot shape fabrication method. Ten other studies in this review investigated the effect of using in-shoe pressure measurement analysis to guide the fabrication of the footwear and insole.[34] The use of a data-driven approach for insole and footwear design has been heralded as authenticating plantar foot pressure reduction on an individual basis. Identification of the vulnerable plantar areas with pressure mapping, in conjunction with foot shape, can help guide the design of personalized footwear and insoles to more effectively reduce the risk of pressure ulceration.

Material Type

The material used, dependent on its intrinsic mechanical properties, will influence the insole or footwear's ability to redistribute or dampen forces effectively. The review found no consistency with individual materials used or thickness in the construction of footwear or insole. The most common insole base material was ethylene vinyl acetate (EVA) with the hardness of 50°–55° Shore A and 30°–35° Shore A. the medium density EVA base (30°–35° Shore A) insoles showed improved performance in offloading peak plantar pressures but needed more frequent replacement than the higher density EVA group insoles because of material fatigue. PPT and/or Poron urethane foam as mid-layer in conjunction with top cover materials such as MCR, plastozote, or microfiber were found to be effective in plantar forefoot pressure reduction. However, the use of a leather top cover was of limited benefit because of its poor pressure reduction capacity.[34]

SHOE MODIFICATIONS

Most diabetic neuropathic patients will benefit from a Depth inlay shoe which is composed of soft leather or composite that will accommodate for toe deformity and volume fluctuations with its high toe box. Extra-depth also allows the addition of orthotics and other modifications. In-shoe orthotic inlays have been shown to be effective in preventing ulceration as assessed by a Cochrane review.[35] The purpose of modifications is to further adapt the footwear and insole for more effective targeted pressure relief. Three key modifications include extra-depth footwear, metatarsal additions, and sinks and apertures. The inability to distinguish the effect of individual modifications from other insole and design features for most studies creates uncertainty on their effectiveness in the prevention of pressure ulcers. Despite this limitation, meta-analyses verified the positive effect of metatarsal pad, cutouts, or apertures in reducing forefoot plantar pressures. It is important to note that the effectiveness in reducing plantar pressure varies considerably with the placement of the pad. One study established a pattern of increases or decreases in metatarsal plantar pressure according to the placement of the metatarsal pad proximal or distal to the metatarsal head, although only the effect on the second metatarsal head was studied.[36]

CUSTOMIZED ORTHOTIC INSOLES FOR RETAIL FOOTWEAR

Suitably designed customized footwear has been proven to reduce forefoot plantar pressures and the risk of re-ulceration. However, poor adherence to customized insoles especially total contact casted and depth inlay shoes is a key barrier to clinical success especially in diabetic individuals without a history of ulceration because they may not consider themselves at risk. For individuals at risk of ulceration but unwilling or unable to change their footwear, an orthotic insole used inside a retail shoe may still offer some protection against the risk of ulceration. One study focused on pressure-relieving orthotic insoles designed for retail footwear in diabetics at risk for forefoot ulceration. The aim was to investigate whether the pressure-relieving effects of a customized metatarsal bar and forefoot cushioning are sensitive to bar location and shape, and material choice in retail footwear. Patient-specific foot shape was used to design an orthotic insole, with metatarsal bar location and shape customized according to plantar pressure data recorded using an instrumented platform while the subject stood. A set of nine customized orthotic insoles were designed to investigate changes in forefoot plantar pressure when people with diabetes and neuropathy walked in nine variants of the orthotic insole. The most frequent reductions in plantar pressure occurred when the anterior edge of the metatarsal bar was placed at 77% of the peak pressure values, and its effects were independent of the choice of overlying offloading material. These results demonstrate that kinetic informed-based fabrication of insoles can be applied to retail footwear for patients who are noncompliant with other options to reduce their risk of ulceration.[37]

DESIGN PROTOCOL FOR CUSTOM-MADE FOOTWEAR FOR DIABETIC PATIENTS

Custom-made footwear is often prescribed to people with diabetes who are at risk for ulceration but are not good candidates for over-the-counter depth inlay shoes. Despite the available scientific evidence and options, there is no uniform evidence-based protocol that is widely used by clinicians to help them select specific footwear design features tailored to their individual patients. One study aimed to develop a design protocol to support custom-made footwear prescriptions for people with diabetes and peripheral neuropathy. A group of experts from rehabilitation medicine, orthopedic shoe technology (pedorthics), and diabetic foot research, reviewed the scientific literature and convened during 12 face-to-face meetings to develop a footwear design algorithm and evidence-based pressure-relief algorithm. Consensus was reached where evidence was not available. Fourteen domains of foot pathology in combination with loss of protective sensation were specified for the footwear design algorithm and for each domain shoe-specific and insole (orthosis)-specific features were defined. These algorithms should help facilitate more uniform decision-making in the prescription and manufacturing of custom shoes for moderate-to-high-risk patients, reducing variation in footwear provision and improving clinical outcomes in the prevention of diabetic foot ulcers.[38]

FUTURE DIRECTIONS
Data-Driven Custom-Made Footwear

The greatest challenge in creating appropriate shoe modifications is in evaluating the actual forces that lead to tissue breakdown to accurately place the modifications for the optimal decrease in plantar pressures. Unfortunately, patient feedback is inadequate due to the presence of neuropathy. Most often, a trial-and-error approach with subsequent inspection of the feet is typically used. More objective methods to evaluate the footwear, such as in-shoe plantar pressure analysis, are not regularly used in the clinic, although this may be most effective at reducing plantar pressures. In a recent study, dynamic in-shoe plantar pressure distribution was measured in 23 neuropathic diabetic foot patients wearing fully customized footwear. Regions of interest with elevated peak pressures were targeted for pressure optimization via shoe modifications. After making modifications, the effect of in-shoe plantar pressure was measured, and mean peak pressure was subsequently reduced in many of these regions. These findings suggest that in-shoe plantar pressure analysis is an effective and efficient tool to evaluate and guide footwear modifications that significantly reduce pressure in the neuropathic diabetic foot and thereby decrease the risk for the development of diabetic pressure injuries.[39] Another study assessing the effect of data-driven custom-made footwear concepts on plantar pressure relief to prevent diabetic foot ulceration showed significantly reduced metatarsal head peak pressure compared with the non-therapeutic shoe condition (17%–53% relief).[40]

Intelligent Insoles

One prospective, randomized study investigated the effectiveness of an intelligent insole system (designed to measure static plantar pressure continuously during daily activities and guide regular self-directed, dynamic offloading) in preventing diabetic foot ulcers in people with diabetes at high risk of ulcer development. The study reported a 71% reduction in ulcer incidence when using the "intelligent" insoles compared with the control group. The study shows that plantar pressures might be able to be used as a feedback signal to compensate for the loss of sensation because of diabetic peripheral neuropathy and help to prevent foot ulcer recurrence.[41]

SUMMARY

Diabetic individuals with peripheral neuropathy are at risk for the development of foot ulcers because of musculoskeletal abnormalities and abnormal loading in the gait cycle leading to elevated plantar pressures. To prevent diabetic foot ulcers, practitioners should regularly screen for presence of neuropathy as well as neuroarthropathies and prescribe the appropriate shoes and orthotics based on the best available clinical evidence. Although not widely available, there is potential for data-driven customization of orthotics and shoe wear based on plantar pressure data to prevent the development of diabetic foot ulcers more effectively and ultimately amputations.

CLINICS CARE POINTS

- An important aspect of preventing diabetic foot ulcers is patient education. It is imperative to counsel the diabetic patient on smoking cessation and adequate glycemic control to prevent peripheral vascular disease and peripheral neuropathy. It is recommended to perform an annual screen for loss of protective sensation using the Semmes–Weinstein monofilament test.

- A slower walking velocity is associated with lower plantar pressures as the vertical ground reaction force increases with faster walking velocities.

- It is important to increase the softness and cushioning of the insole to evenly distribute plantar pressures, which supplements the function of the fat pads that can atrophy with age and neuropathy. By conforming to the shape of the foot, this allows a reduction in pressure by increasing the area over which the force is applied.

- A rigid outsole or shank can reduce metatarsophalangeal and tarsometatarsal joint dorsiflexion in the stance phase and thereby reduce pressure concentration under the metatarsal heads and strain on the plantar ligaments.
- In-shoe plantar pressure analysis is an effective and efficient tool to evaluate and guide footwear modifications that significantly reduce pressure in the neuropathic diabetic foot and thereby decrease the risk for the development of diabetic pressure ulcers.

DISCLOSURE

The authors have nothing to disclose.

REFERENCES

1. Mason J, O'Keeffe C, Hutchinson A, et al. A systematic review of foot ulcer in patients with type 2 diabetes mellitus. II: treatment. Diabet Med 1999;16(11): 889–909.
2. Reiber GE, Lipsky BA, Gibbons GW. The burden of diabetic foot ulcers. Am J Surg 1998;176(2 A):5S–10S.
3. Mcneely MJ, Boyko EJ, Ahroni JH, et al. The independent contributions of diabetic neuropathy and vasculopatny in foot ulceration: How great are the risks? Diabetes Care 1995;18(2):216–9.
4. Apelqvist J, Agardh CD. The association between clinical risk factors and outcome of diabetic foot ulcers. Diabetes Res Clin Pract 1992;18(1):43–53.
5. Olmos PR, Cataland S, O'Dorisio TM, et al. The Semmes-Weinstein monofilament as a potential predictor of foot ulceration in patients with noninsulin-dependent diabetes. Am J Med Sci 1995;309(2):76–82.
6. Hicks JH. The mechanics of the foot. II. The plantar aponeurosis and the arch. J Anat 1954;88(1):25–30. Available at: http://www.ncbi.nlm.nih.gov/pubmed/ 13129168%0Ahttp://www.pubmedcentral.nih.gov/articlerender.fcgi?artid=PMC 1244640.
7. Perry J. Anatomy and biomechanics of the hindfoot. Clin Orthop Relat Res 1983; 177:9–15.
8. Boulton AJM, Whitehouse RW. The Diabetic Foot. [Updated 2020 Mar 15]. In: Feingold KR, Anawalt B, Boyce A, et al, editors. Endotext [Internet]. South Dartmouth (MA): MDText.com, Inc.; 2000.
9. Armstrong DG, Lavery LA, Harkless LB. Validation of a diabetic wound classification system: The contribution of depth, infection, and ischemia to risk of amputation. Diabetes Care 1998;21(5):855–9.
10. Eid MA, Mehta KS, Goodney PP. Epidemiology of peripheral artery disease. Semin Vasc Surg 2021;116:1509–26.
11. Boyko EJ, Ahroni JH, Stensel V, et al. A prospective study of risk factors for diabetic foot ulcer: The seattle diabetic foot study. Diabetes Care 1999;22(7):1036–42.
12. Bus SA, Yang QX, Wang JH, et al. Intrinsic muscle atrophy and toe deformity in the diabetic neuropathic foot: a magnetic resonance imaging study. Diabetes Care 2002;25(8):1444–50.
13. Gilbey SG, Walters H, Edmonds ME, et al. Vascular calcification, autonomic neuropathy, and peripheral blood flow in patients with diabetic nephropathy. Diabet Med 1989;6(1):37–42.

14. Kimura T, Thorhauer ED, Kindig MW, et al. Neuropathy, claw toes, intrinsic muscle volume, and plantar aponeurosis thickness in diabetic feet. BMC Musculoskelet Disord 2020;21(1). https://doi.org/10.1186/s12891-020-03503-y.
15. Mann RA. Pathological anatomy of claw and hammer toes. J Bone Joint Surg Am 1990;72(2):305.
16. Bus SA. Foot structure and footwear prescription in diabetes mellitus. Diabetes Metab Res Rev 2008;24(SUPPL. 1). https://doi.org/10.1002/dmrr.840.
17. DiPreta JA. Metatarsalgia, lesser toe deformities, and associated disorders of the forefoot. Med Clin North Am 2014;98(2):233–51.
18. Grant WP, Sullivan R, Sonenshine DE, et al. Electron microscopic investigation of the effects of diabetes mellitus on the achilles tendon. J Foot Ankle Surg 1997; 36(4):272–8.
19. Arangio GA, Chen C, Salathé EP. Effect of varying arch height with and without the plantar fascia on the mechanical properties of the foot. Foot Ankle Int 1998; 19(10):705–9.
20. Giacomozzi C, D'Ambrogi E, Uccioli L, et al. Does the thickening of Achilles tendon and plantar fascia contribute to the alteration of diabetic foot loading? Clin Biomech 2005;20(5):532–9.
21. Bellary S, Anwar AJ, Harvey TC. The Charcot foot. Lancet 2003;361(9364):1225.
22. Sanders L, Frykberg R. Diabetic neuropathic osteoarthropathy: the Charcot foot. In: Robert G Fryberg, editor. The high risk foot in diabetes mellitus. New York, 1990: Churchill Livingstone; 1991. p. 297–338.
23. Reiber GE, Smith DG, Vileikyte L, et al. Causal pathways for incident lower-extremity ulcers in patients with diabetes from two settings. Diabetes Care 1999;22(1):157–62.
24. Allet L, Armand S, de Bie RA, et al. Gait alterations of diabetic patients while walking on different surfaces. Gait Posture 2009;29(3):488–93.
25. Zimny S, Schatz H, Pfohl M. The role of limited joint mobility in diabetic patients with an at-risk foot. Diabetes Care 2004;27(4):942–6.
26. Kwon OY, Mueller MJ. Walking patterns used reduce forefoot plantar pressures in people width diabetic neuropathies. Phys Ther 2001;81(2):828–35.
27. Burnfield JM, Few CD, Mohamed OS, et al. The influence of walking speed and footwear on plantar pressures in older adults. Clin Biomech 2004;19(1):78–84.
28. Reiber GE, Smith DG, Wallace CM, et al. Footwear used by individuals with diabetes and a history of foot ulcer. J Rehabil Res Dev 2002;39(5):615–21.
29. van Netten JJ, Lazzarini PA, Armstrong DG, et al. Diabetic Foot Australia guideline on footwear for people with diabetes. J Foot Ankle Res 2018;11(1). https://doi.org/10.1186/s13047-017-0244-z.
30. Collings R, Freeman J, Latour JM, et al. Footwear and insole design features for offloading the diabetic at risk foot—A systematic review and meta-analyses. Endocrinol Diabetes Metab 2021;4(1). https://doi.org/10.1002/edm2.132.
31. Tsung BYS, Zhang M, Mak AFT, et al. Effectiveness of insoles on plantar pressure redistribution. J Rehabil Res Dev 2004;41(6 A):767–74.
32. Nawoczenski DA, Birke JA, Coleman WC. Effect of rocker sole design on plantar forefoot pressures. J Am Podiatr Med Assoc 1988;78(9):455–60.
33. Schaff PS, Cavanagh PR. Shoes for the insensitive foot: the effect of a "rocker bottom" shoe modification on plantar pressure distribution. Foot Ankle Int 1990; 11(3):129–40.
34. Ahmed S, Barwick A, Butterworth P, et al. Footwear and insole design features that reduce neuropathic plantar forefoot ulcer risk in people with diabetes: A

systematic literature review. J Foot Ankle Res 2020;13(1). https://doi.org/10.1186/s13047-020-00400-4.

35. Spencer SA. Pressure relieving interventions for preventing and treating diabetic foot ulcers. Cochrane Database Syst Rev 2000;3. https://doi.org/10.1002/14651858.cd002302.

36. Hastings MK, Mueller MJ, Pilgram TK, et al. Effect of metatarsal pad placement on plantar pressure in people with diabetes mellitus and peripheral neuropathy. Foot Ankle Int 2007;28(1):84–8.

37. Martinez-Santos A, Preece S, Nester CJ. Evaluation of orthotic insoles for people with diabetes who are at-risk of first ulceration. J Foot Ankle Res 2019;12(1). https://doi.org/10.1186/s13047-019-0344-z.

38. Bus SA, Zwaferink JB, Dahmen R, et al. State of the art design protocol for custom made footwear for people with diabetes and peripheral neuropathy. Diabetes Metab Res Rev 2020;36(S1). https://doi.org/10.1002/dmrr.3237.

39. Bus SA, Haspels R, Busch-Westbroek TE. Evaluation and optimization of therapeutic footwear for neuropathic diabetic foot patients using in-shoe plantar pressure analysis. Diabetes Care 2011;34(7):1595–600.

40. Zwaferink JBJ, Custers W, Paardekooper I, et al. Optimizing footwear for the diabetic foot: Data-driven custom-made footwear concepts and their effect on pressure relief to prevent diabetic foot ulceration. PLoS One 2020;15(4). https://doi.org/10.1371/journal.pone.0224010.

41. Abbott CA, Chatwin KE, Foden P, et al. Innovative intelligent insole system reduces diabetic foot ulcer recurrence at plantar sites: a prospective, randomised, proof-of-concept study. Lancet Digit Heal 2019;1(6):e308–18.

Post Amputation Skin and Wound Care

Michael Kwasniewski, MD[a],*, Danielle Mitchel, MD[b],[1]

KEYWORDS

- Amputation • Residual limb • Dysvascular • Dehiscence • Prosthetic or prosthesis

KEY POINTS

- Although there is no consensus in the literature regarding dressing choice and wound care for patients with amputations, the most appropriate dressing for the postamputation wound is tailored to the patient's specific wound care needs.
- An appropriate postoperative dressing provides moisture at the incision line conducive to healing, management of edema that may slow the process, and protection of the limb from trauma and contracture.
- Some small, descriptive studies show there may be some superiority of rigid dressings over soft dressings; however, rigid dressings pose additional integumentary risks to a patient with multiple comorbidities, which entails the majority of patients with amputation.
- Most common dressing for postoperative lower limb amputations: nonadherent dressing on the incision, sterile gauze 4 × 4s, rolled gauze holding the prior two in place, and a compression wrapping.
- Regular inspection of the surgical incision allows for early detection and treatment for skin breakdown, wound dehiscence, infection, and contracture.

INTRODUCTION

The care of a postoperative patient with amputation in the rehabilitation setting is multifaceted and requires coordination of care from the surgical team, physiatrist, physical and occupational therapists, nursing, and wound care specialists. With regards to the management of the surgical wound postoperatively, the approach varies by provider. The literature review reveals very few articles of good quality delineating what is first-line wound care for a patient with amputation. Additionally, most of the studies conducted only involve transtibial amputations, without the involvement of transfemoral or any upper extremity amputations. In this article, we have attempted to

[a] Inpatient Amputation Rehabilitation Program, MossRehab, 60 Township Line Road, Elkins Park, PA 19027, USA; [b] Physical Medicine and Rehabilitation, Temple University Hospital/ MossRehab, 3401 N. Broad Street, Lower Level, Rock Pavilion, Philadelphia, PA 19140, USA
[1] Present address: 60 Township Line Road, Elkins Park, PA 19027.
* Corresponding author.
E-mail address: michael.kwasniewski@jefferson.edu

Phys Med Rehabil Clin N Am 33 (2022) 857–870
https://doi.org/10.1016/j.pmr.2022.06.010
1047-9651/22/© 2022 Elsevier Inc. All rights reserved.

pmr.theclinics.com

provide a basis of how to care for the surgical wound of a new patient with amputation from the postoperative period into outpatient, with an understanding that what follows is based more on general consensus in clinical experience than highly substantiated evidence.

Definition of terms	
Terms	**Definitions**
Contracture	A deformity at a joint that develops from persistent shortening of muscles/tendons/joints[1]
Eschar	A type of necrotic tissue that adheres to the wound bed. Typically dark or black in color.[2]
Epithelialization	A process during wound healing where epithelial cells migrate up in the wound bed to repair the damaged area.[3]
Granulation tissue	A complex connective tissue comprised of fibroblasts, keratinocytes, endothelial cells, capillaries, and extracellular matrix that forms at the site of a wound to function as the building blocks for wound healing and future epithelization.[4]
Gangrene	The death of a tissue secondary to lack of oxygenation (commonly because of infection or peripheral arterial disease).[5]
Slough	A type of necrotic tissue that does not adheres to the wound bed. Typically yellow or white in color.[6]
Shrinker	An elastic sock made intentionally for compression of a residual limb.
Wound dehiscence	The partial or complete separation of previously approximated wound edges.[7]

PHYSIOLOGY OF WOUND HEALING

On a molecular level, wound healing in a healthy individual is organized into three overlapping phases: inflammation, proliferation, and maturation/remodeling. This cascade of events is sometimes referred to as "the inflammatory process" as it is mediated by inflammatory cytokines.[8] We now provide a basic overview of the phases.

Phase 1: Inflammation

The first phase of wound healing occurs from the start of injury to about five days postinjury. This is both a vascular and cellular response. The blood vessels near the site of injury initially leak transudate causing tissue edema, which results in decreased pressure in the vessels, slowing blood loss. Multiple types of cells migrate to the site to control blood loss, fend off bacteria, and activate the process of tissue repair.

Phase 2: Proliferation

This phase starts around the 2-day postinjury mark until about 2 weeks. During this phase, new tissues build into the gap to fill and close the wound. Processes occurring at this time include angiogenesis (the formation of new blood vessels), the formation of granulation tissue, wound contraction, and epithelialization. Note that eschar and slough must be removed while trying to keep granulation tissue intact for epithelialization to occur.

Phase 3: Maturation and Remodeling

Maturation occurs from 2 weeks until about 2 years postinjury in healthy individuals. This final phase is what allows scar tissue to reorganize to achieve its maximal potential for strength and function. Collagen at this time is remodeled rather than built upon. Of important note, once fully healed, a scar can only reach 80% of a tissue's original strength, at best.

INTENTION HEALING OF SURGICAL WOUND CLOSURES

Different types of wound closures, or "intentions" can affect the healing of a wound and are important to note when trying to optimize healing. There are three intentions—primary, secondary, and tertiary—that indicate distinct types of healing taking place (**Table 1**). Postamputation surgical incisions may exhibit one or more of these closures, which may require the physician to change the type of dressing used.

PATIENT EVALUATION

When assessing the surgical incision after an amputation, it is important to expose the entire incision and visualize the surrounding skin. Take note of any edema, abnormal color change, and bruising of the surrounding skin. Next, assess the wound edges for approximation versus any areas of wound dehiscence. Inspect the wound and any open areas for the presence of granulation tissue, eschar, and slough. Take note of drainage and any purulence. In the overall examination of the patient, assess vital signs and any signs or symptoms indicating infection or excessive pain. All of these factors contribute to the selection of appropriate wound dressings to create the optimal environment for healing.

COMORBIDITIES

Overall, the two main causes of amputation in the United States are vascular disease (54%) and trauma (45%); the remaining amputations are due to congenital deformities, cancer, and so forth.[9] Among those with lower limb amputations, dysvascular disease accounts for 82%.[10] Therefore, a majority of patients with an amputation will have multiple comorbidities, including diabetes, hypertension, peripheral vascular disease, renal disease, and obesity. These comorbidities factor heavily into the most common reasons for amputation, including nonhealing wounds, osteomyelitis, and gangrene. Just as these conditions present a challenge to the healing of any wound, an

Table 1
Comparison of wound closure classifications

Wound Closure Classification		
Primary	**Secondary**	**Tertiary**
Clean incision—trauma or surgery	Significant tissue loss, ulceration, pressure, burns	Contaminated wounds that require cleaning & monitoring or dehisced wounds
Wound edges well approximated for closure	Poor approximation with gapping	Delayed primary closure when clean
Closure with sutures or staples	Closure by formation of granulation tissue	Vacuum-assisted closure may help expedite healing
Rapid healing, minimal granulation and scarring	Daily dressing changes, high granulation	Subsequent healing by primary or secondary closure

amputation is no exception. Following an amputation, it is critical to control these comorbidities to promote the best chance for healing without complications. Strict control of blood sugar, blood pressure, electrolytes, and nutrition maximize healing potential. This often requires close collaboration between the rehab provider, endocrinologists, nephrologists, registered dieticians, and cardiologists.

Additionally, modifiable risk factors, such as cigarette smoking and recreational drug use, impact the body's ability to heal. Practitioners should strongly emphasize cessation of these activities and offer psychological and/or pharmacological support.

GOALS OF POST AMPUTATION WOUND CARE

For the patient with amputation, there are goals for both the healing of the surgical site and for rehabilitation. The dressing needs to maintain a balanced, moist environment for the wound itself. To prevent maceration, the best environment for healing is one that has moisture at the incision line but is dry at the surrounding healthy tissue. The dressing should promote healing by first or second intention, prevent microorganisms from entering the wound, absorb drainage, and remove necrotic tissue if it appears.

From a functional perspective, the dressing should be able to support early mobilization and rehabilitation to expedite advancement to prosthetic fitting. Ideally, the dressing should keep the limb in extension to help prevent/minimize contracture, preserve range of motion, and provide some degree of protection. The outer component of the dressing should provide compression to facilitate ideal shaping of the residual limb.

WOUND DRESSINGS
Overview

Dressings for the postamputation surgical wound vary widely at the incision level and in the materials with which they are wrapped. At the incision level, the goal is to achieve a moisture-balanced environment; too much fluid in a wound bed can cause the skin and underlying tissues to macerate, while too dry a wound can slow epithelial migration to the area and impair healing. Thus, it is important to tailor the dressing to the patient's wound and keep a close eye on the skin to modify the dressing over time. Most wounds do best with a moist environment while keeping the surrounding intact skin dry. Once the agent for direct contact with the incision is chosen, then the next step is to decide how to adhere that agent to the wound bed, be it through occlusive or semiocclusive dressing. The final step is to decide what class of outer dressing is most appropriate for edema control, positioning, and protection of the residual limb.

Step 1: directly cover the incision
Petroleum-based, nonadherent mesh gauze. A petroleum-based, nonadherent dressing is a common choice to promote a moist healing environment in drier surgical wounds. The two most frequently used brands are Xeroform and Adaptic. Xeroform is a sterile mesh gauze saturated with a mix of 3% bismuth tribromo-phenate and petroleum. It is best for dry and nonexudative wounds as it maintains an appropriately moist environment and may provide some antibacterial coverage.[11] Adaptic is a sterile mesh gauze saturated with petroleum that is also nonadherent to the wound. Used for a wider spectrum of surgical incisions, Adaptic is indicated for dry to highly exudative wounds. Moisture is maintained while being able to absorb exudate and allow excess to pass through to the secondary dressing.[12]

Gelling fiber. Another type of dressing is a gelling fiber, which is typically constructed of a cellulose structure that forms a gel when in contact with exudate. The gel traps fluid, keeping it from re-entering the dressing or affecting nearby healthy tissue, making it a good choice for moderate to heavy exudative wound.[13] Gelling should not be used for dry wounds as it would further dehydrate the wound bed and impair healing.

Sterile packing. Sometimes the surgical amputation wound can dehisce, which can happen along the entire incision or only in limited areas. When dehiscence is small along the suture line, but the opening is deep, sterile packing is the appropriate dressing choice. Sterile packing allows for the absorption of exudate from within a wound, allowing it to heal from the inside.[13] Without packing, the wound may heal superficially at the top without filling in with granulation tissue appropriately. Two types of commonly used packing are plain sterile packing or iodoform packing, the latter saturated with an iodoform solution that has antibacterial properties.

Vacuum-assisted closure. Wounds where a larger portion of the suture line or the entire suture line has become dehisced require notification and recommendations from the surgeon who performed the amputation. In some cases, they may determine that a vacuum-assisted closure (VAC) for the wound is appropriate. A wound VAC provides negative pressure to the wound bed, increasing blood flow, accelerating the formation of granulation tissue, decreasing edema, and promoting lymphatic drainage, all while pulling together the wound edges.[14]

Step 2: secondary dressing

Occlusive dressings. Transparent dressings, often made of polyurethane, are adhesive semipermeable membranes that act as a barrier against outside bacteria.[15] They allow for visualization of the wound as well as autolytic debridement. They are primarily for superficial wounds or as secondary dressings over dressings, such as alginates/hydrogels, that allow for rehydration of the wound bed.[2] However, because they do not allow the outflow of exudate, they can put nearby healthy tissue at risk of maceration. Additionally, they are adhesive to the neighboring tissues, and in patients with amputation who have multiple comorbidities, the daily or twice daily changing of an adhesive dressing may be abrasive to nearby tissue, causing new damage beyond the surgical incision. For such reasons, they are not the first line choice for amputation wounds.

Dry dressing. These include cotton, wool, natural/synthetic bandages, and gauze. These dressings are dry and do not promote a moist environment, which is suboptimal for healing wounds that are dry at the onset. They have some utility in exudative wounds but need to be changed regularly to avoid maceration of underlying tissue. While they can serve as the primary dressing choice, sterile gauze bandages and/or rolls are more commonly used to secure the primary dressing in place and to capture any breakthrough exudate.

Step 3: outer dressing—compressive and protective

There is no significant consensus on what is the most effective outer dressing for the postamputation residual limb. The studies that exist in the literature are mostly descriptive, with low numbers of participants, low power, and no universal outcome measure. Types of wrapping dressings are soft, semirigid, and rigid, with further subcategories of immediate postoperative prosthesis (IPOP), and prefabricated pneumatic postoperative prosthesis. The most commonly used is the soft dressing for its low cost, ease of application, and accessible view of the surgical incision. One of the only randomized trials comparing soft dressings to rigid dressings was done in 1977; that study found a shorter time from surgery to initial gait training with a rigid dressing but did not find a difference in healing rates of soft versus rigid dressings.[16]

Additionally, that study did not adjust its statistical analysis for comorbidities. In other small descriptive comparison studies, there was no statistically significant difference in the rate of falls, length of hospitalizations, or reduced mortality with rigid versus soft dressings.[17–19] We briefly review descriptions of each dressing type in the following sections.

Soft
- Typically consists of a nonadherent dressing on the incision, sterile gauze 4 × 4's, rolled gauze holding the prior two in place
- Can be used without or with compression wrapping, the latter being more often utilized
- Benefits: Allows for easy inspection of the residual limb so that wound issues can be addressed promptly.
- Risks: Less compression compared to other methods, may lead to slower healing
- Most common overall, though training for appropriate compression and wrapping style with elastic bandage is an important part of postoperative management for the patient
- Compression wrapping is required to control postoperative edema
  - Note that compression cannot be so significant that it pulls on the incision in such a way to encourage dehiscence
  - An elastic bandage (ie, ACE wrap) or elastic tubular bandage (ie, Tubigrip) is most commonly used over the soft dressing.
  - If using an elastic bandage wrap, then the residual limb should be rewrapped in a figure-of-eight configuration at least every 6 hours to ensure adequate and even compression (**Fig. 1**).
  - A shrinker (**Fig. 2**) is not typically indicated until the surgical wound is healed, as the donning of a shrinker places unwanted shear forces on an unhealed incision that could result in dehiscence.

Semirigid
- Utilizing Unna Boot bandages (gauze saturated in zinc oxide or calamine lotion), applied without pressure and shrinks while drying
- Benefits: Provides better compression for edema management than soft dressing as well as some degree of protection of the wound
- Risks: Less frequent ability to inspect skin. Not indicated in patients who are insensate, have neuropathy, or patients at risk of pressure injuries.[20]
- Allow for skin checks every 3+ days, but generally applied by a professional

Rigid
- The residual limb is wrapped in a rigid plaster cast, either removable (**Fig. 3**) or nonremovable
- Benefits: May decrease time from amputation to preparatory prosthesis, good control of edema, and decreased risk for contracture
- Risks: Delay in identifying wound issues, increased risk for pressure injuries
- Newer prefabricated versions of rigid removable dressings not requiring casting are continuing to be evaluated.
- May be more feasible for young trauma patients with intact sensation who want to be ambulatory as soon as possible, but risky for patients with known/suspected healing issues and/or who are insensate
- Variations
  - IPOP (**Fig. 4**)

- Rigid cast with a pylon and foot attached so that patient can immediately being gait training with partial weight bearing
- Although uncommon, could mostly be used for young patients with great healing potential who have good balance and skin tensile strength
- Not indicated for dysvascular patients or those with comorbidities that will impair healing[21]
  ○ Prefabricated pneumatic postoperative prosthesis (**Fig. 5**)
- A hard socket lined with air cells; attached pylon and prosthetic foot
- Placed over soft dressing, can be inflated/deflated to apply compression
- Similar to an IPOP, allows for partial weight bearing soon after surgery
- Feasibility study showed comparable wound complications to patients with soft/rigid postoperative dressings[22]
- Require expert to don/doff device

AMPUTEE REHABILITATION TIMELINE

Immediately postoperatively, the patient will don one of the aforementioned dressings as deemed appropriate by their surgeon. Ideally, upon discharge from the hospital, the patient will enter acute inpatient rehabilitation or subacute rehabilitation for preprosthetic training. At this time, a physiatrist will take over, directing wound care as the incision heals and evolves. The medical focus is on wound and skin monitoring and healing, edema management, pain control, and managing comorbidities. From the therapy perspective, the focus is on maintaining range of motion, preventing contracture, promoting early mobilization, cardiovascular fitness, and functional mobility training. They will continue to dress the wound as dictated by the discharging

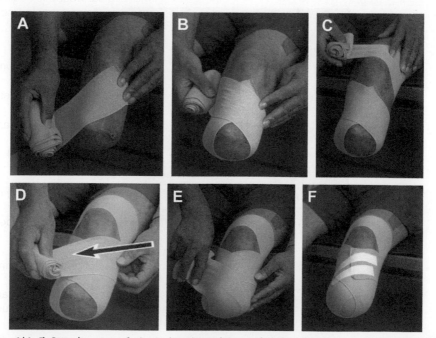

Fig.. 1(*A–F*) Step by step of elastic bandage figure-of-eight wrapping configuration with anchoring above the knee in a patient with a transtibial amputation.

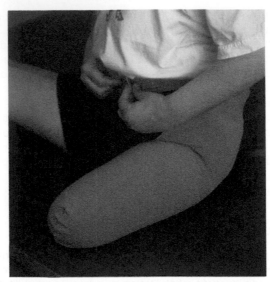

Fig. 2. Compressive shrinker donned on a patient with healed transfemoral amputation.

physician until the postoperative visit with the surgeon. When the patient's surgeon gives clearance that the surgical wound is healed (often 4–8 weeks post-op), the patient will transition to the use of a shrinker for limb shaping. The shrinker is to be donned at all times, with the exception of bathing. With optimized healing and limb

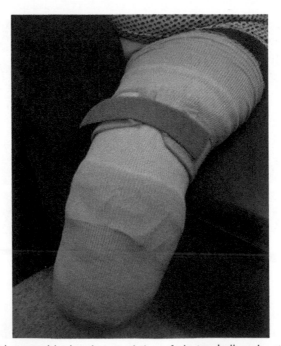

Fig. 3. Classic rigid removable dressing consisting of plaster shell, socks, stockinette tubular dressing, and supracondylar cuff.

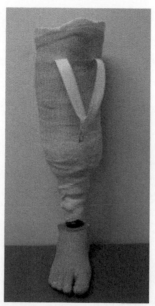

Fig. 4. IPOP with prosthetic foot.

shaping, generally around 2–3 months from the date of surgery, the physiatrist will pre-scribe the appropriate preparatory prosthesis. After the prosthesis has been fitted and use is initiated, skin management remains important to prevent any potential skin breakdown and the development of other wounds.

POSTOPERATIVE SKIN COMPLICATIONS IN PERSONS WITH AMPUTATIONS
Infection

Infection is unfortunately a common complication of amputation. There are currently no large meta-analyses giving a clear picture of what percentage of amputations are found to be infected during the course of healing; descriptive and retrospective studies estimate 17%–40% of major lower limb amputations have reported infec-tions.[15] Patients with amputations and comorbidities, such as diabetes, malnutrition, malignancy, peripheral arterial disease, cigarette smoking, and so forth are at an increased risk of developing infection. Clinically, it is important to be vigilant in the postoperative period, regularly evaluating the wound, surrounding skin, and patient as a whole. Erythema, warmth, unexplained increases in pain, purulent drainage, dehiscence of the wound, poor wound healing, and fever should trigger concern for infection. In one study of 231 patients, the most common pathogens infecting ampu-tation wounds were methicillin-resistant *Staphylococcus aureus*, *Pseudomonas aeru-ginosa*, Enterococcus, *Escherichia coli*, *Proteus mirabilis*, and *Klebsiella pneumoniae*.[15] For suspected cellulitis, empirical prophylactic antibiotic therapy can be started with ciprofloxacin, cefalexin, or clindamycin. If infection persists or it ap-pears deep rather than superficial, it may require prompt surgical evaluation for possible irrigation and debridement of the wound.

Adhesion

Postoperative adhesions occur most frequently at bony prominences and at areas of scarring. For patients with lower extremity amputations, this can be common at the

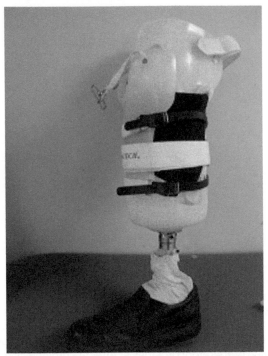

Fig. 5. Pneumatic postoperative prosthesis with plastic shell and air cells for fit.

distal end of the long bones. If skin grafting was required for limb management, these areas were also more prone to developing adhesions. Adhesions can become problematic in the postoperative phase, but more so with prosthetic fitting as skin may be more prone to wound development if it is not able to move well. As such, skin mobilization is important both at the incision line and in the surrounding skin as early as post-op day 1. Early post-op technique includes approximation of the suture line and gentle skin movement. Subsequent management with transverse friction massage and myofascial release once the incision is healed and well approximated. All these techniques are managed as part of the therapy regimen for patients following amputation.

Contracture

As mentioned earlier, when dressing the residual limb, it is important to maintain nearby joints in extension to prevent the formation of contractures. A contracture is a deformity at a joint that develops from persistent shortening of muscles/tendons. Once a contracture forms, it may not be possible to fully resolve it with therapy or surgery, so prevention is key. Regarding skin and wound management, contracture prevention is most important if skin grafting or surgical incisions cross any joint lines. Measures, such as educating the patient not to put a pillow under the joint, encouraging supine exercises for lower limb amputees, and performing regular range of motion exercises in therapy can help prevent and resolve contractures as they are starting to form.

Wound Dehiscence

A phenomenon where the wound edges separate completely is called wound dehiscence. Although not as common as infection, one study of 287 amputee patients found a dehiscence rate of 16%.[23] Treatment in a rehabilitation center may be possible; however, when the entire wound dehisces, surgical intervention is likely. Underlying factors that cause dehiscence include infection, hematoma, and comorbidities that impair wound healing (ie, diabetes, smoking, malnutrition, obesity). For partial dehiscence, the surgeon may recommend trying a wound VAC, as discussed in the section titled, "Vacuum-assisted closure." Wounds that fail wound VAC management will require further surgical evaluation.

PAIN ETIOLOGIES

Although pain does not directly affect wound healing, it can secondarily play a factor in wound and skin management and/or be a symptom indicative of another underlying issue. As such, it should be managed appropriately.

Nociceptive

Acute pain from surgery is expected in the first 1 to 3 weeks postoperatively. Pain that worsens or extends beyond the acute period should be investigated. Some causes of excessive pain in the residual limb include hematoma, dehiscence, infection, and heterotopic ossification. The formation of a hematoma at the distal residual limb can result in significant discomfort and pain as well as delayed wound healing with further potential complications of wound dehiscence or provide a nidus for infection. Postoperative bleeding that is persistent can require reoperation in 3%–9% of major lower limb amputations.[24] In contrast, heterotopic ossification is a rare early complication of amputation, where abnormal bone growth leads to bone deposition in soft tissues. Although rarely factored into primary wound healing, further interventions may be required in the future for management. A radiograph of the residual limb or a triple phase bone scan assist in identifying this complication, which may require involvement of endocrinology and treatment with a bisphosphonate medication.[25] Other etiologies, such as neuroma, bursitis, or tendonitis of the residual limb should be considered.

Neuropathic or Phantom

Phantom or neuropathic pain also requires appropriate management to aid in wound and skin management. Often described as tingling, burning, cold, numbness, or electric sensation,[26] the incidence of immediate postoperative phantom pain is reportedly 70%–80%, whereas incidence at 6 months ranges from 60% to 90%.[27] Although neuropathic pain does not directly impact the surgical wound or wound healing, related hypersensitivity and/or allodynia can impact the ability to provide adequate skin and wound management and necessary edema control. Lack of appropriate edema management can subsequently lead to undue stress on the surgical wound and delay healing or potentially result in dehiscence.

REAMPUTATION

The amputation wound requires close observation because the rates of surgical revision after major amputation remain high. In one study of over 3500 dysvascular patients, 26% required secondary amputation procedures within 12 months of initial major lower extremity amputation.[28] One study of diabetic patients showed rates of reamputation in diabetic patients to be 26.7% at 1 year, 48.3% at 3 years, and 60.7% at 5 years.[29] Causes for reamputation include ischemia in the residual limb, necrosis developing in the wound bed (ie, presence of eschar), dehiscence, infection, and persistently nonhealing surgical incision. Detection of any of these issues should trigger prompt notification of the patient's surgeon for further evaluation. In one review of over 8800 amputees at various levels, the risk factors independently associated with initial amputation failure included the following: age > 80 years, emergency operation (ie, guillotine amputation), end stage renal disease, systemic inflammatory response syndrome, obesity, and ongoing tobacco use.[30]

EVALUATION OF LONG-TERM OUTCOMES

Overall, an optimized and shorter time to healing results in a higher likelihood of prosthetic use for improvement of function. Functional outcomes are associated with skin healing and vary based on many factors, including level of amputation, etiology, preoperative functional status, medical comorbidities, and the patient's network. A survey of traumatic amputation patients using the Sickness Impact Profile found that "patient characteristics that were significantly associated with poorer outcomes included older age, female gender, nonwhite race, lower education level, living in a poor household, current or previous smoking, low self-efficacy, poor self-reported health status before the injury, and involvement with the legal system in an effort to obtain disability payments."[31] In terms of transition to prosthetic usage after amputation, one study found that rates of prosthetic use range from 27% to 56% in upper limb amputations and 49%–95% in lower limb amputations.[32] Early and appropriate postamputation skin and wound management is an important driver in restarting a move back toward functional independence.

SUMMARY

Postoperative wound care in the patients with amputation is an individualized process that evolves as the patient heals. As there is no consensus in the literature for a clear standard of care, the same type of wound may be treated successfully with different styles of dressings. An appropriate postoperative dressing wrapped in soft gauze and compression bandage is the most commonly used, given that a majority of nontraumatic patients with amputation have comorbidities that preclude them from safely using a rigid dressing. Regular inspection of the incision, adapting the dressing as the incision heals, managing comorbid conditions and common postoperative complications, and keeping the patient's surgeon involved will lead to prompt detection and treatment of issues as they arise.

DISCLOSURE

The authors have nothing to disclose.

REFERENCES

1. Muscle contracture and stiffening symptoms. UPMC. UPMC Orthopaedic Care; 2021. Available at: https://www.upmc.com/services/orthopaedics/conditions-treatments/contractures-and-stiffness. Accessed October 4, 2021.
2. Klein LJ. Evaluation of the hand and upper extremity. Cooper's Fundamentals of Hand Therapy (Third Edition). Available at: https://www.sciencedirect.com/science/article/pii/B9780323524797000041. Accessed October 4, 2021.
3. Tan ST, Dosan R. Lessons from epithelialization: the reason behind Moist Wound Environment. Open Dermatol J 2019;13(1):34–40.
4. Alhajj M, Bansal P, Goyal A. Physiology, granulation tissue. In: StatPearls. Treasure Island (FL): StatPearls Publishing; 2021. Available at: https://www.ncbi.nlm.nih.gov/books/NBK554402/.

5. Clinic Mayo Staff. Gangrene. mayo clinic. Available at: https://www.mayoclinic. org/diseases-conditions/gangrene/symptoms-causes/syc-20352567. Accessed October 4, 2021.
6. Grey JE, Enoch S, Harding KG. Wound assessment. BMJ 2006;332(7536):285–8.
7. Rosen RD, Manna B. Wound dehiscence. In: StatPearls. Treasure Island (FL): StatPearls Publishing; 2021. Available at: https://www.ncbi.nlm.nih.gov/books/ NBK551712/.
8. Kumar V, Abbas A, Aster J. Robbins basic pathology E-Book. Saint Louis: Elsevier; 2017. Chapter 4: Tissue Repair.
9. Pasquina PF, Miller M, Carvalho AJ, et al. Special considerations for multiple limb amputation. Curr Phys Med Rehabil Rep 2014;2(4):273–89.
10. Cifu D, Cifu D, Braddom R. Braddom's physical medicine and rehabilitation. 6th edition. Elsevier; 2020. Chapter 10: Lower Limb Amputation.
11. Barillo DJ, Barillo AR, Korn S, et al. The antimicrobial spectrum of Xeroform. Burns 2017;43(6):1189–94.
12. WoundSource. 3M™ Adaptic™ Non-Adhering Dressing. 2021 [online] Available at: https://www.woundsource.com/product/3m-adaptic-non-adhering-dressing. Accessed 4 October 2021.
13. Nagy K. Discharge instructions for wound cares. the american association for the surgery of trauma. 2013. Available at: https://www.aast.org/resources-detail/ discharge-instructions-wound-cares. Accessed October 4, 2021.
14. Zayan NE, West JM, Schulz SA, et al. Incisional negative pressure wound therapy: an effective tool for major limb amputation and amputation revision site closure. Adv Wound Care (New Rochelle) 2019;8(8):368–73.
15. de Godoy JM, Ribeiro JV, Caracanhas LA, et al. Hospital infection after major amputations. Ann Clin Microbiol Antimicrob 2010;9:15. Available at: https://doi-org. libproxy.temple.edu/10.1186/1476-0711-9-15.
16. Smith D, McFarland L, Sangeorzan B, et al. Postoperative dressing and management strategies for transtibial amputations: a critical review. J Prosthetics Orthotics 2004;16(Supplement):S15–25.
17. Mooney V, Harvey J, McBride E, et al. Comparison of postoperative stump management. J Bone Joint Surg 1971;53(2):241–9.
18. Wu Y, Keagy R, Krick H, et al. An innovative removable rigid dressing technique for below-the-knee amputation. J Bone Joint Surg 1979;61(5):724–9.
19. Schon L, Short K, Soupiou O, et al. Benefits of early prosthetic management of transtibial amputees: a prospective clinical study of a prefabricated prosthesis. Schon et al. Foot Ankle Int 2002;23:509–14.
20. Conde Montero E. Bandages impregnated with zinc oxide: Unna boot and much more. Dr. Elena Conde MD, PhD. Dermatologist. 2020. Available at: https://www. elenaconde.com/en/bandages-impregnated-with-zinc-oxide-unna-boot-and-much-more/. Accessed October 4, 2021.
21. Boucher HR, Schon LC, Parks B, et al. A biomechanical study of two postoperative prostheses for transtibial amputees: a custom-molded and a prefabricated adjustable pneumatic prosthesis. Foot Ankle Int 2002;23(5):452–6.
22. Pinzur MS, Angelico J. A feasibility trial of a prefabricated immediate postoperative prosthetic limb system. Foot Ankle Int 2003;24(11):861–4.
23. Dunkel N, Belaieff W, Assal M, et al. Wound dehiscence and stump infection after lower limb amputation: risk factors and association with antibiotic use. J Orthop Sci 2012;17(5):588–94.
24. Kalapatapu V. UpToDate. Uptodate.com. 2021. Available at: https://www. uptodate.com/contents/lower-extremity-amputation?search=lower%20extremity

%20amputation&source=search_result&selectedTitle=1~80&usage_
type=default&display_rank=1. Accessed October 4, 2021.

25. Abrams G, Wakasa M. Chronic complications of spinal cord injury and disease. UpToDate. 2021. Available at: https://www.uptodate.com/contents/chronic-complications-of-spinal-cord-injury-and-disease?search=heterotopic%20ossification&sectionRank=1&usage_type=default&anchor=H18&source=machineLearning&selectedTitle=3~34&display_rank=3#H18.   Accessed October 4, 2021.

26. Kaur A, Guan Y. Phantom limb pain: a literature review. Chin J Traumatol 2018; 21(6):366–8.

27. Standard of care: lower extremity amputation. Brigham and Women's Hospital. 2021. Available at: https://www.brighamandwomens.org/assets/BWH/patients-and-families/rehabilitation-services/pdfs/general-le-amputation-bwh.pdf.   Accessed October 4, 2021.

28. Dillingham TR, Pezzin LE, Shore AD. Reamputation, mortality, and health care costs among persons with dysvascular lower-limb amputations. Arch Phys Med Rehabil 2005;86(3):480–6.

29. Izumi Y, Satterfield K, Lee S, et al. Risk of reamputation in diabetic patients stratified by limb and level of amputation: a 10-year observation. Diabetes Care 2006; 29(3):566–70.

30. O'Brien PJ, Cox MW, Shortell CK, et al. Risk factors for early failure of surgical amputations: an analysis of 8,878 isolated lower extremity amputation procedures. J Am Coll Surg 2013;216(4):836–42 [discussion: 842-4].

31. MacKenzie EJ, Bosse MJ, Pollak AN, et al. Long-term persistence of disability following severe lower-limb trauma. Results of a seven-year follow-up. J Bone Joint Surg Am 2005;87(8):1801–9.

32. Raichle KA, Hanley MA, Molton I, et al. Prosthesis use in persons with lower- and upper-limb amputation. J Rehabil Res Dev 2008;45(7):961–72.

An Introduction to Burns

Sarah Ashouri, MSN, CRNP*

KEYWORDS

- Burn • Burn dressings • Burn care • Introduction to burn

KEY POINTS

- Burn care improvements across time have drastically improved mortality rates.
- Many avenues of wound care exist for burn treatment, but none replace surgical excision.
- Early excision and grafting are the "gold standard" of burn care.
- New methods of autografting have revolutionized the care of patients with large burn injuries.
- Physical Medicine and Rehab (PM&R) enables the patient to advance their quality of life.

INTRODUCTION

The American Burn Association (ABA) defines burn injury as damage to the skin and underlying tissues resulting from heat, chemicals, or electric sources.[1] Burn injury remains a significant source of morbidity in the United States impacting 400,000 to 450,000 victims per year.[1,2] Victims of burn injury are often left with life-altering sequelae after recovery.

Historic documentation revealed archaic burn wound treatment consisted largely of topical ingredients such as cattle dung, vinegar, onion, tea leaf extracts, and animal fat.[3–5] Operative intervention surfaced with the introduction of early surgical excision by Ambroise Pare, but it was soon deserted due to the inability to obtain hemostasis, the inability to replenish blood volume, post-excision site infections, and the inability to sterilize surgical instruments.[4,5] Wound care, though poorly understood at the time, encouraged the sloughing of eschar and thus continued as the mainstay of treatment.[4] Unfortunately, limitations in treatment along with a lack of pathophysiologic understanding of burn injury and roaring infections[4,5] made burn victims more likely to perish than not.

In the spirit of standardization, Dr Hildanus of Germany developed the burn depth classification system in 1634 that eventually transitioned into the classification system we use today.[4] Lister began sterilizing surgical instruments in 1865 thus improving postoperative infections and mortality.[5] Burn resuscitation changed during World

Trauma Burn Surgery, University of Alabama at Birmingham, 9601, NP 9th Floor, 1802 6th Avenue South Birmingham, AL 35233, USA
* Corresponding author.
E-mail address: sarahashouri@uabmc.edu

Phys Med Rehabil Clin N Am 33 (2022) 871–883
https://doi.org/10.1016/j.pmr.2022.07.001

War II as plasma infusion was introduced as a substitute for whole blood.[6] World War II also provided mathematical resuscitation formulas that considered the victim's burn size and weight.[6] Soon after, early excision was recognized as a valuable intervention in reducing burn mortality[5] though it only became widely accepted in the 1970s when Zora Janzekovic introduced tangential excision.[4,5]

Autografting was first described by the Indian surgeon Sushrutha in the fifth century as a treatment for the wounds of criminals whose noses were amputated as a punishment.[4,5] Pieces of skin were rotated downward from the forehead to cover the nasal defect, beginning the practice of tissue mobilization.[4,5] Bunger furthered this practice by using full-thickness pieces of tissue from the donor's thigh to cover a nasal defect in 1823.[4,5] Unfortunately, graft failure as a result of infection and excessively thick grafts resulted in a high failure rate.[4,5]

In 1869, Reverdin transplanted "pinch grafts" to wound beds which resulted in quick wound epithelialization in both the donor site and autograft site.[4,5] Blair and Brown discovered that donor skin could be harvested at varying depths as long as deep islands of hair follicles and sebaceous gland epithelial cells were preserved, thus leading to the development of the adjustable dermatome and subsequent popularization of split-thickness skin grafting (STSG).[4,5] The challenge of optimizing wound coverage was addressed by the development of the Meek micrografting technique, which was soon followed by the skin mesher, both of which focused to expand skin for optimal wound coverage.[4,5] Unfortunately, in patients with a large total body surface area (TBSA) burn, wound coverage remained a concern. This inspired the use of cadaveric skin for temporary closure.[4] With the dramatic change in burn care over the last 100 years came to a significant reduction in mortality of the burn patient.[7]

The goal of this article is to provide the nonburn specialized reader with a brief insight into burn care, briefly discuss current advances in burn care, and present the role of Physical Medicine and Rehab (PM&R) in the recovery of burn patients.

INITIAL MANAGEMENT

Burn care begins at the moment of injury with the primary survey which is then followed by the secondary survey.[1,8–10] Preliminary estimation of burn size, beginning resuscitation, stopping the burning process, removing the patient and caregiver from harm's way, and timely transportation to a burn center are crucial steps in mobilizing the care of an acutely burned patient.[1,8,10]

To optimize survival, the primary survey is designed to efficiently address immediate threats to life and limb at the first point of contact with the injured victim.[1] It is used in both trauma and burn life support curriculums to rapidly evaluate the condition of the airway ("A"), the patient's breathing ("B"), their circulation ("C"), if they have any disabilities ("D") (neurologic), and what they have been exposed to in the environment ("E").[1] The acronym "ABCDE" is an easy way to remember the sections of the primary survey in order.[1]

Airway and breathing are often assessed simultaneously. The patient is assessed for their current and anticipated ability to maintain their airway.[1] Signs such as facial burns, singed nasal passages, presence of soot in the oropharynx and nasal passages, vocal hoarseness,[11,12] and stridor along with the occurrence of the burn event in an enclosed space are often indications of inhalation injury.[11–13] Full-thickness injuries of the head and neck may warrant escharotomies to avoid compartment syndrome and loss of the victim's airway.[14] Cervical spine protection should always be maintained until cervical collar can be safely cleared.[1]

Circulation is assessed using heart rate and rhythm, blood pressure, skin color, and warmth of the skin.[1] Care should be taken not to miss less obvious injuries that may be insulting the patient's physiology resulting in hypovolemic shock.[1] The expectation is that burn patients with large burns have two large bore intravenous catheters (IVs) and initial fluid rates begun per Advanced Burn Life Support curriculum guidelines.[1]

Assessing disability necessitates evaluation of alertness ("A"), ability to respond to verbal stimulation ("V") versus painful stimulation ("P"), or if the patient is unresponsive ("U") using "AVPU" in addition to the use of the Glasgow Coma Scale.[1] Completely undressing the patient for a full physical evaluation, removing all nonadherent items such as shoes and jewelry, and stopping the burning process to ensure minimization of the insult is also expected at this time.[1] Ensuring a warm environment and putting dry coverings on the victim after the primary survey reduces the risk of hypothermia.[1,8]

The secondary survey follows the primary survey and functions to ensure all injuries and baseline facts about the burn victim are known. Circumstances surrounding the incident, patient's medical history ("AMPLET"), preinjury weight, full-body physical (including burn severity, depth, and extent (rule of nines and/or palmar method)) should be acquired.[1] Fluids should be shifted from initial rates to adjusted rates. Resuscitation continues as the providers monitor urine output (UOP), vital signs, and compartment pressures.[1] Pain and anxiety should be managed via IV route with opioids and/or benzodiazepines.[1] Serum labs and imaging should be obtained at this time.[1]

An institution is designated as a burn center when they possess the resources necessary to provide comprehensive care to the burn patient. The ABA has delineated extensive criteria addressing competency in all aspects of the burn care which must be met and authenticated via review and site visit for a facility to be considered a verified burn center.[15] A burn center may exist and provide burn care without being an ABA verified burn center, though verification through this rigorous review is a sign of excellence and should be sought after. Given the specialized nature of burn centers, the ABA has developed criteria for referral (**Box 1**) to streamline which patients should be referred to a burn center.[16]

Box 1
ABA criteria for burn center referral[16]

Greater than 10% TBSA partial-thickness burns

Burns of the face, hands, feet, genitalia, perineum, or major joints

Full-thickness burns

Electrical burns (includes lightning injury)

Chemical burns

Inhalation injury

Burn injury in patients with preexisting medical disorders that may complicate burn management, prolong their recovery time, or influence mortality.

Patients with burns and traumatic injury in which the burn poses a greater risk of morbidity or mortality. If the trauma poses a greater immediate risk, the patient may be initially stabilized in a trauma center before being transferred to a burn unit.

Burned children in hospitals without qualified personnel of equipment for the care of children.

Burn injury in patients who require special social, emotional, or long-term rehabilitative intervention.

INJURY SEVERITY, BURN SHOCK, AND RESUSCITATION

To estimate burn size, there are several methods that may be used. Examples include The Lund Browder diagram, the Rule of Nines, and the Palmar Method. A comparison of TBSA estimation methods is outlined in **Table 1**.

The Lund Browder method is generally more accurate whereas the Rule of Nines is less accurate but easier and faster to use.[1] For children, the Rule of Nines is inaccurate.[17] The Palmar method is fastest for small burns or burns which are scattered and can be used by estimating the patient's palm and fingers as 1% TBSA[1] though this is inaccurate in an obese or cachectic patient.[17] Erythematous areas (first degree) are not included in the TBSA calculation regardless of what method is used to assess.[1]

When considering injury severity, the victim's age, wound depth, and TBSA are taken into consideration. Of note, greater than 20% TBSA in adults, greater than 10% TBSA in children and the elderly, and greater than 5% TBSA full-thickness burns, high voltage burn, or chemical burns to face, eyes, ears, genitalia, or major joints, or clinically significant trauma constitutes a major burn and warrants referral to a burn center.[14,17] A severely injured burn patient should be resuscitated and monitored in an ICU with nurses and providers who are experienced in burn resuscitation. Acutely, a burn victim having sustained $\geq$20% TBSA shows a pathophysiologic response referred to as burn shock.[18] Burn shock is manifested by soft-tissue edema, intravascular volume depletion, cardiac depression, and increased systemic vascular resistance.[19–21]

In brief, inflammatory mediators (eg, histamines, prostaglandins, bradykinin, angiotensin II, vasopressin, and thromboxane) and elevated nitric oxide levels are activated by the large burn injury resulting in vascular luminal endothelial dysfunction resulting in "leaky capillaries" from oxidative stress.[17,19] Intravascular proteins then shift extravascularly into the interstitium. As a result, the patient experiences a decrease in intravascular colloid osmotic pressure as the patient's plasma volume shifts toward the newly displaced protein, thus engorging both the injured and uninjured interstitial space (a phenomenon known as "third spacing").[19,20] Cardiac depression, increased afterload, and decreased cardiac contractility occur as a result of a multitude of factors including circulatory mediators and impaired Ca^{+2} utilization at the cellular level.[20] To treat burn shock, a multitude of burn resuscitation formulas exist with the more popular ones being Evans Formula, Brooke formula, modified Brooke Formula, and Parkland Formula (**Table 2**).[18,30]

Of note, children, the elderly, and those with inhalation injuries have different fluid requirements.[18] Resuscitation is largely guided by UOP with a goal of 75 to 100 mL/h for burn patients with an electrical injury and 0.5 mL/kg/h for other mechanisms.[1,17] Serum lab values should also be used to gauge the patient's resuscitative direction.[18] Resuscitation remains an art in the burn community. Over-resuscitation puts the patient at risk for abdominal compartment syndrome, pulmonary edema, extremity compartment syndrome, and cerebral edema,[18] and death. Similarly, under-resuscitation puts the patient at risk for organ failure and death as well.[22] Although the mainstay of burn shock treatment remains fluid resuscitation, therapeutic plasma exchange and hemofiltration have shown some promise in attenuating the inflammatory response that incites burn shock.[17]

BURN EVALUATION, CLASSIFICATION, AND MECHANISM OF INJURY

First-degree burns are superficial, painful, and do not blister. They injure the epidermis only. Examples include many sunburns and some flash burns.[23] Second-degree burns are also known as partial-thickness burns. They are defined as burns in which the

Table 1
Comparison of TBSA estimation methods[14]

Name of Method	Head	Neck	Trunk	Arms	Legs	Genitals	Buttocks
			Percent TBSA Allocation				
Lund Browder	7%–19% age dependent	1% front 1% back	13% front 13% back	5% front 5% back	5%–9.75% age dependent	1%	2.5% each
Rule of Nines	4.5% front 4.5% back	Included with head	18% front 18% back	4.5% front 4.5% back	9% front 9% back	1%	Included with legs
Palmar Method	The size of the patient's palm and fingers equals 1% TBSA.						

Table 2 Comparison of resuscitation formulas[18,30]	
Formula Name	Formula
Parkland	4 mL LR x kg x % TBSA Give ½ in the first 8 h. Give ½ in the subsequent 16 h. Colloid after second 24 h.
Brooke	2 mL x kg x TBSA; 0.5 mL/kg per TBSA given as colloid, 1.5 mL/kg per TBSA given as crystalloid.
Modified Brooke	2 mL x kg x TBSA, colloid use after second 24 hrs.
Evans	1 mL x kg x TBSA of NS. And an equal part colloid plus 2000 mL D5W

injury extends through the epidermis to the dermis. If the injury extends through the superficial dermal layer, it is coined superficial partial thickness. These burns are painful, pink, have a quick capillary refill, and are blistered.[14,24] Deep partial thickness burns extend into the deep layer of the dermis and show varying sensation, have capillary refill (though it may seem a slightly delayed), are often pale pink or have a mottled pink and white appearance, and may have hemorrhagic blisters.[14] Full-thickness burns show damage that extends beyond the dermis and require excision and grafting. They initially present as painless, leathery to the touch, and are often white or brown. Burns that are not anticipated to heal within 21 days often benefit from grafting. Superficial burns often heal well with proper wound care and dressing changes. Despite the availability of many modes of evaluation such as biopsy, thermography, vital dye injection, and laser Doppler techniques, clinical observation remains the standard.[25]

When evaluating wounds and anticipating progression, the mechanism of injury is important to take into consideration. Thermal injuries include flash burns, flame burns, chemical burns, electrical injuries, scalds, and contact burns.[26] Flash burns may cover large areas and often impact the skin that is not protected with clothing as well as the upper airway.[26] Luckily, flash burns often heal with minimal grafting unless the clothing caught on fire.[26] A victim whose clothes have caught on fire suffers from intense heat for a prolonged period of time which often results in deep dermal or full-thickness burns that may require grafting.[26]

Chemical burns differ depending on the offending agent. Burns in which the offending agent is acidic (pH <7) typically create a "tan" that prevents further penetration of the chemical resulting in a superficial, self-limiting injury.[26] Alkali burns (pH >7) are typically more severe since alkalotic substances combine with adipose tissue to create soap, a reaction that continues until it is neutralized or severely diluted with water as occurs with decontamination.[26]

Electrical injuries are categorized as low voltage (<440 V) or high voltage (1000 V). Low voltage burn wounds typically have few sequelae beyond deep burn wounds at contact points. High voltage burn wounds are associated with deep tissue damage. Injury to smaller body parts such as fingers, hands, and forearms may require emergent decompression with escharotomies, fasciotomies, and carpal tunnel release. Early operative intervention (<3 days from injury) is recommended if the patient is not clearing a lactic acidosis or myoglobinuria with standard resuscitation protocol.[26]

Scalds result in wounds of varying depth depending on the type of liquid and exposure time.[26] Thicker liquids (such as sauces, grits, and porridge) and liquids that are absorbed by clothing often create deep dermal burns as a result of prolonged exposure to the skin.[26] Hot oils often create deep dermal and full-thickness burns that may require skin grafting because of the intense amount of energy required to heat them.[26] Of note, it is imperative to watch for immersion scalds in special populations such as the elderly and the youth as this may be a sign of abuse.[26]

Contact burns result from skin making contact with a hot object.[26] Wound depth depends on the temperature of the object and the duration of contact.[26] The degree of devastation is varying and may be anywhere from partial thickness to full thickness extending through the fat and down to the muscle.[26] Especially important are combination crush and burn injuries that often require immediate intervention because of compartment syndrome and myonecrosis.

WOUND CARE

Hydrotherapy is a mode of cleansing the patient on a waterproof table. This allows for optimal wound care as the patient may be easily positioned and cleansed. Novel approaches to hydrotherapy continue to emerge including collaboration with anesthesia to offer advanced pain control during this painful procedure.

Burn dressings are important in providing comfort, moisture, fluid loss control, and decreasing the patient's pain. The initial contact layer should be nonadherent and is where any antibiotic is found. An absorbent layer follows, functioning to pull fluid away from the wound. The dressing is then secured with a snug-fitting outer wrap.

Dressings can be divided into short-term and long-term types. Short-term dressings are dressings that must be changed daily. This includes ointments, creams, debriding agents, and soak dressings. Triple antibiotic ointment, Bacitracin, Silver Sulfadiazine, mupirocin ointment, Dakin's solution, silver nitrate, mafenide acetate, and amphotericin B soaks are all included in this category. Triple antibiotic ointment provides wide antimicrobial coverage and may be used on the face and neck as it does not cause staining. However, prolonged use may result in hypersensitivity and drug concentrations do not treat infection.[27]

Bacitracin provides narrow bacterial coverage, mostly gram-negative microorganisms. It provides a moist wound environment and is typically used for small wounds and facial burns. Silver sulfadiazine provides broad-spectrum antibacterial coverage, but has been shown to delay re-epithelialization and stain tissues. As such, its use on the face and neck is avoided. It is often associated with the development of a pseudoeschar that may be painful to remove. Patients with a sulfa allergy may develop an allergic reaction and it is known to cause a transient neutropenia in some patients.[28] Mupirocin ointment provides coverage of gram-positive organisms, but is often expensive. Since it does not cause staining, it is also an option for use on the face and neck.

Dakin's solution is a liquid hypochlorite antiseptic that has been used since World War I when it revolutionized infection control.[29] It is available in various strengths (0.025%, 0.25%, and 0.5%) and is applied directly to the gauze dressing every 4 to 6 h, thus "soaking" the wound. Strengths greater than 0.025% are thought to show high cytotoxicity.[27,29] Silver nitrate solution functions to provide broad antibacterial coverage without the risk of graft toxicity though it may cause electrolyte imbalances.[27] Mafenide acetate is available in both a cream and solution. It provides broad-spectrum antimicrobial coverage with low cytotoxicity. However, it may cause metabolic acidosis and is often painful for patients.[30] Mafenide acetate cream penetrates eschar well and is effective on the ears and nose.[30] Amphotericin B soaks are used on patients exhibiting fungal infection[27] and are often alternated with an additional soaks dressing such as mafenide acetate.

Long-term dressings, often silver infused, can be applied to a clean wound and left in place for 5 to 7 days. Often recommended for partial-thickness burns, their ease of use makes them favorable among burn care providers and the lack of daily dressing changes tends to decrease pain for the patient. Many brands exist though one has not proven better over the other. The silver in the dressings may discolor wounds or cause a delay in healing.

With many options available, the decision of which dressing to pursue may be intimidating. Luckily, key situational characteristics often make it easier to choose. Wounds requiring serial evaluations, that are overwhelmed with biofilm, have embedded debris, or are in areas of the body that are frequently soiled (such as near or on genitalia) benefit from daily and/or as needed dressing changes as opposed to long-term dressing application. Wounds that are partial thickness, stable, free of biofilm, and thought to be at low risk for infection and soiling are often good options for long-term dressings. Patients who do not qualify for home health nursing and have little social support and are unable to perform their own dressing changes often benefit from long-term dressings as well.

OPERATIVE INTERVENTIONS

Before operative intervention, comorbid conditions such as diabetes should be optimized. Mobility and nutrition should be preoperatively evaluated and optimized as well. Given the hypermetabolic response induced by burn injury, it is imperative that nutrition is carefully maintained throughout the patient's hospitalization by trending serum prealbumin, providing a protein-rich diet with protein supplementation, and supplemental tube feeds if needed.[30]

Early excision and grafting, though variable in definition and long a topic of debate, is the "gold standard" of treatment[30] and has been shown to reduce mortality and hospital length of stay. Invariably, the excision of deeper wounds may reveal underlying structures such as tendon or bone, which may require the application of a dermal substitute to granulate the wound. Once granulated and ready, the wound is autografted for closure.[30,31]

Autografting remains the mainstay of wound closure in the burn world.[30,32,33] Cutaneous autografting exists as split-thickness skin grafting (STSG) or full-thickness skin grafting (FTSG).[34] STSG extends the depth of the epidermis and a portion of the dermis, whereas the depth of the FTSG extends through the entirety of the dermis.[34] Harvesting of an FTSG requires subsequent primary closure.[34] Split thickness autografts leave behind a portion of the dermis, thus allowing epithelialization.of the donor site.[34] Unfortunately, in the case of a larger burn wound, autografting creates more open wounds in the form of donor site that ultimately increase the open TBSA.

Luckily, newer technologies exist such as cultured epithelial autograft (CEAs) and autologous skin cell suspension (ASCS) which have revolutionized burn care—particularly in the setting of patients lacking donor sites.[17] CEAs are cultured cells grown in a lab after the patient's sample is received.[35] Challenges posed by CEAs include the length of time waiting for skin to grow and long-term fragility.[17,36] It is also very expensive.[17] ASCS requires that a donor site is harvested and the cells processed through an enzymatic solution that separates them, rinsed with a buffer solution, filtered, and ultimately transformed into a liquid suspension which is then sprayed over meshed autograft in the case of excised full-thickness wounds.[32] As the ASCS can also be applied to wounds with healthy dermis to hasten healing, it can be applied to donor sites for faster re-epithelialization as well.[37] Healing time is shown to be faster with the use of ASCS.[17] This method has revolutionized the autografting of burn patients with a large TBSA injury who lack donor sites as well as the care of cosmetically important areas such as the face.[32,38]

Allograft, the use of cadaveric donor skin for temporary wound closure, remains widely used for several reasons. Cryopreservation of donor skin provides a biological dressing with a long shelf-life resulting in a product that can be kept for an extended period of time.[28] Allograft vascularizes when applied and remains adherent to the wound bed until rejection (typically 3–4 weeks after application)[28] and is proposed to decrease fluid and heat loss as well as improve healing.[24]

Xenograft, nonviable porcine skin, has been used in the past as a biologic dressing. It was applied directly to debrided partial-thickness burns and STSG donor sites to decrease pain, hasten healing, and protect the wound interstices of STSG in a "sandwich" technique.[39] Unfortunately, porcine xenograft is no longer produced and is now unavailable.

REHABILITATION

Many sequelae of burn injury exist. Hypertrophic scarring, scar contracture, heterotopic ossification (HO), loss of mobility, and pain are commonly part of the aftermath of a burn injury. PM&R plays a vital role in the recovery and the quality of life (QOL) of the burn patient. PM&R focuses on the preservation and restoration of mobility, activities of daily living (ADLs), limb positioning, splinting, and scar management as common parts of the patient's treatment plan.[17] Physical therapists (PTs) and occupational therapists (OTs) are often introduced to the burn patient early on in their course and continue to follow throughout their burn care journey.[17]

Hypertrophic scarring can be defined as the occurrence of thick, inelastic scar tissue which is raised above the level of the skin and does not extend beyond the margins of the original wound.[40,41] The pathophysiology of hypertrophic scarring is not fully understood.[42] However, it is thought that it may develop as a result of the absence of typical apoptotic activity of myofibroblasts as a consequence of prolonged wound healing ultimately resulting in excessive collagen deposition in the extracellular matrix.[42] Hypertrophic scarring often presents in the first 1 to 3 months following injury[40] with a prevalence of as much as 70%.[26] Hypertrophic scarring remains a challenge for patients and clinicians alike and is known to decrease QOL as a consequence of continued itching, pain, and change in appearance.[40,42] Treatment begins with a thorough scar assessment which would include the use of a hypertrophic scarring rating tool such as the Vancouver Scar Scale (VSS) or the Patient and Observer Assessment Scale (POSAS) as well as documentation of the percentage of the raised area of healed wound.[40] The use of compression garments, silicone, corticosteroid injections, exercise, pulsed light therapy, and scar massage are treatment modalities that are widely used in the burn world though more rigorous studies on the efficacy of these treatments are needed.[41,43,44]

Scar contracture may also be detrimental to the burn survivor's QOL because of limitations in mobility which may impair the performance of ADLs.[45] Treatment often includes surgical intervention for which there is a lack of strong methodological data thus warranting further study.[46]

Silicone, available in various forms, is a mainstay of burn scar treatment. It is painless, easy to apply, and effective.[41] It is appreciated for its moisturizing and occlusive properties which decrease neurogenic inflammation and pruritus.[42] It is recommended that silicone be worn 12 to 24 h per day for several months.[40] Compression garments have been described as early as the 1800s and are thought to influence the collagen remodeling phase of healing.[40,41] They are recommended to be worn at least

23 h per day with a pressure of 24 to 40 mm Hg.[40,41] Unfortunately, pressure garments show limited effectiveness at the joints, are often costly, are not attractive, and can be difficult to apply resulting in low patient compliance.[40]

HO is the formation of bone in soft tissues thought to be associated with the inflammatory response of the burn injury.[17,47,48] Particularly devastating is the development of HO of the joint. It is most often seen in the elbows where it results in a decrease in mobility and may result in ulnar nerve entrapment[25] HO is associated with increased hospital length of stay, pain, distress, significantly reduced joint mobility, and nerve entrapment.[25] Unfortunately, the cellular mechanisms have not yet been established.[25] As a result, no clear guidelines for prevention exist. Treatment regimens have previously included aggressive occupational therapy though this remains controversial.[48]

Continued pain often exists for burn patients for a prolonged period after their wounds have healed and is often associated with scarring.[49] Prolonged pain influences all areas of life including emotion, and ADLs. The etiology of continued pain remains unclear, though it is thought to be related to the release of inflammatory mediators which influence the peripheral nerves.[50] Current treatments include mainstay scar therapies such as lasers and compression in addition to oral analgesics, elevation, and rest.[48] Unfortunately, the pain often continues for a prolonged period of time.[48] Given the pain and other sensory alterations, there is a need for additional research on sensory changes in post-burn wounds.[51]

CLINICS CARE POINTS

- Burn care has advanced significantly in the last 100 years with a drastic decrease in mortality as a result.
- The primary and secondary surveys as detailed by the Advanced Burn Life Support Curriculum lay the foundation for subsequent burn care.
- Patients who meet the American Burn Association referral criteria should be referred to a burn center for evaluation
- Various methods exist to calculate total body surface area. The Lund Browder method is the most accurate and takes into consideration victim age.
- Various resuscitation formulas exist and resuscitation protocol is often facility-specific.
- Injury severity differs based on age and injury.
- Burns should be evaluated and treated by an experienced burn provider.
- Early excision and autographing remains the "gold standard".
- Various wound care methods exist.
- Physical Medicine and Rehab significantly increases the quality of life of the burn patient post-injury.

DISCLOSURE

The author has nothing to disclose.

REFERENCES

1. Pham, T. N., Bettencourt, A. P., Bozinko, G. M., et al (2017). 2018 ABLS Provider Manual 1.

2. Crowe CS, Massenburg BB, Morrison SD, et al. Trends of burn injury in the United States 1990 to 2016. Ann Surg 2019;270(6):944–53.

3. MLK. Branski, DN. Herndon, RE. Barrow. A Brief History of Acute Burn Care Management. Total Burn Care, edited by David N. Herndon. University of Texas Medical Branch, 2018. Available at: https://www-sciencedirect-com.ezproxy3.lhl.uab.edu/science/article/pii/B9780323476614000010. Accessed May 3, 2022.

4. Lee KC, Joory K, Moiemen NS. History of burns: The past, present and the future. Burns Trauma 2014;2(Issue 4):169–80.

5. Liu HF, Zhang F, Lineaweaver WC. History and advancement of burn treatments. Ann Plast Surg 2017;78(Issue 2):S2–8.

6. Gurney JM, Kozar RA, Cancio LC. Plasma for burn shock resuscitation: is it time to go back to the future? Transfusion 2019;59(S2):1578–86.

7. El Khatib A, Jeschke MG. Medicina contemporary aspects of burn care. Medicina 2021;57(4):386. https://doi.org/10.3390/medicina57040386. Available at: Accessed May 4, 2022.

8. Allison K, Porter K. Consensus on the prehospital approach to burns patient management. Emerg Med J 2004;21(1):112–4.

9. Alonso-Fernández JM, Lorente-González P, Pérez-Munguía L, et al. Analysis of hypothermia through the acute phase in major burns patients: Nursing care. Enfermeria Intensiva 2020;31(3):120–30.

10. Dries DJ. Burn care: before the burn center. Scand J Trauma Resuscitation Emerg Med 2020;28(1). https://doi.org/10.1186/s13049-020-00771-4.

11. Dries DJ, Endorf FW. Inhalation injury: epidemiology, pathology, treatment strategies. Scandinavian Journal of Trauma, Resuscitation and Emergency Medicine 2014;21(1). Available at: http://www.sjtrem.com/content/21/1/31. Accessed June 15, 2022.

12. Walker PF, Buehner MF, Wood LA, et al. Diagnosis and management of inhalation injury: An updated review. Crit Care 2015;19(Issue 1). https://doi.org/10.1186/s13054-015-1077-4.

13. Mlcak RP, Suman OE, Herndon DN. Respiratory management of inhalation injury. Burns 2007;33(1):2–13.

14. Singer AJ, Dagum AB. Current Management of Acute Cutaneous Wounds. N Engl J Med 2008;359(10):1037–46.

15. Palmieri TL, London JA, O'Mara MS, et al. Analysis of admissions and outcomes in verified and nonverified burn centers. J Burn Care Res 2008;29(1):208–12.

16. Carter JE, Neff LP, Holmes JH. Adherence to burn center referral criteria: Are patients appropriately being referred? J Burn Care Res 2010;31(1):26–30.

17. Jeschke MG, van Baar ME, Choudhry MA, et al. Burn injury. Nat Rev Dis Primers 2020;6(1). https://doi.org/10.1038/s41572-020-0145-5.

18. Cancio LC, Bohanon FJ, Kramer GC, Resuscitation Burn. In: Herndon David N, editor. Total Burn Care. University of Texas Medical Branch; 2018. Available at: https://www-sciencedirect-com.ezproxy3.lhl.uab.edu/science/article/pii/B9780323476614000095. Accessed May 3, 2022.

19. Wurzer, P., Culnan, D., Cancio, L. C., & Kramer, G. C. (n.d.). Pathophysiology of Burn Shock and Burn Edema.

20. Latenser BA. Critical care of the burn patient: The first 48 hours. Crit Care Med 2009;37(10):2819–26.

21. Ong YS, Samuel M, Song C. Meta-analysis of early excision of burns. Burns 2006;32(2):145–50.

22. Endorf FW, Dries DJ. Burn resuscitation. Scandinavian Journal of Trauma, Resuscitation, and Emergency Medicine 2011;19(69):1–6. https://doi.org/10.1186/1757-7241-19-69. Available at: Accessed June 20, 2022.
23. Pan SC. Burn blister fluids in the neovascularization stage of burn wound healing: A comparison between superficial and deep partial-thickness burn wounds. Burns Trauma 2013;1(Issue 1):27–31.
24. Leon-Villapalos J, Eldardiri M, Dziewulski P. The use of human deceased donor skin allograft in burn care. Cell Tissue Banking 2010;11(1):99–104.
25. Kornhaber R, Foster N, Edgar D, et al. The development and impact of heterotopic ossification in burns: a review of four decades of research. Scars Burns Healing 2017;3. 205951311769565.
26. Brownson, E. G., & Gibran, N. S. (n.d.). Evaluation of the Burn Wound: Management Decisions.
27. Cambiaso-Daniel, J., Gallagher, J. J., Norbury, W. B., Finnerty, C. C., Herndon, D. N., & Culnan, D. M. (n.d.). Treatment of Infection in Burn Patients.
28. Middelkoop, E., & Sheridan, R. L. (n.d.). Skin Substitutes and "the next level" Temporary Skin Substitutes and Dressings.
29. Georgiadis J, Nascimento VB, Donat C, et al. Dakin's Solution: "One of the most important and far-reaching contributions to the armamentarium of the surgeons. Burns 2019;45(7):1509–17.
30. Roth JJ, Hughes WB. The essential burn unit handbook. 2nd edition. Philadelphia: CRC Press; 2016.
31. Shores JT, Hiersche M, Gabriel A, et al. Tendon coverage using an artificial skin substitute. J Plast Reconstr Aesthet Surg 2012;65(11):1544–50.
32. Holmes JH, Molnar JA, Shupp JW, et al. Demonstration of the safety and effectiveness of the RECELL® System combined with split-thickness meshed autografts for the reduction of donor skin to treat mixed-depth burn injuries. Burns 2019;45(4):772–82.
33. Jeschke MG, Chinkes DL, Finnerty CC, et al. Pathophysiologic response to severe burn injury. Ann Surg 2008;248(3):387–400.
34. ME B, F.M.P. Split-Thickness Skin Grafts. Northwestern Handbook of Surgical Procedures 2019;230–1. https://doi.org/10.1201/b17659-109. Available at: Accessed June 20, 2022.
35. Atiyeh BS, Costagliola M. (n.d.). Cultured epithelial autograft (CEA) in burn treatment: Three decades later. Burns. Vol 33, no 3, pp 40-413. Available at: https://doi.org/10.1016/j.burns.2006.11.002. Accessed June 20, 2022.
36. Wood FM, Kolybaba ML, Allen P (nd. The use of cultured epithelial autograft in the treatment of major burn injuries: A critical review of the literature. Burns 2007;32(4):39–401. https://doi.org/10.1016/j.burns.2006.01.008. Available at: Accessed June 20, 2022.
37. Hu Z, Guo D, Liu P, et al. Randomized clinical trial of autologous skin cell suspension for accelerating re-epithelialization of split-thickness donor sites. British Journal of Surgery 2017;104(7):836–42. Available at: 10.1002/bjs.10508 Accessed June 20, 2022.
38. Molnar JA, Walker N, Steele TN, et al. n.d Initial Experience With Autologous Skin Cell Suspension for Treatment of Deep Partial-Thickness Facial Burns. Journal of Burn Care and Research 2020;41(5). https://doi.org/10.1093/jbcr/iraa037. pp. 104–101 Available at: Accessed June 20, 2022.
39. Chiu T, Burd A. Xenograft" dressing in the treatment of burns. Clin Dermatol 2005;23(4):419–23.

40. Bloemen MCT, van der Veer WM, Ulrich MMW, et al. Prevention and curative management of hypertrophic scar formation. Burns 2009;35(4):463–75.
41. Finnerty CC, Jeschke MG, Branski LK, et al. Burns 2 Hypertrophic scarring: the greatest unmet challenge after burn injury. Lancet 2016;388(1002):1427–36. Available at:www.thelancet.com Accessed June 20, 2022.
42. Chiang RS, Borovikova AA, King K, et al. Current concepts related to hypertrophic scarring in burn injuries. Wound Repair Regen 2016;24(Issue 3):466–77.
43. Gabriel V. Hypertrophic Scar. Phys Med Rehabil Clin North Am 2011;22(Issue 2): 301–10.
44. Tredget EE, Shupp JW, Schneider JC. Scar management following burn injury. J Burn Care Res 2017;38(3):146–7.
45. Oosterwijk AM, Mouton LJ, Schouten H, et al. Prevalence of scar contractures after burn: A systematic review. Burns 2017;43(Issue 1):41–9.
46. Stekelenburg CM, Marck RE, Tuinebreijer WE, et al. A Systematic Review on Burn Scar Contracture Treatment: Searching for Evidence. J Burn Care Res 2015; 36(3):e153–61.
47. Schneider JC, Simko LC, Goldstein R, et al. Predicting Heterotopic Ossification Early after Burn Injuries: A Risk Scoring System. Ann Surg 2017;266(1):179–84.
48. Sun Y, Lin Y, Chen Z, et al. Heterotopic Ossification in Burn Patients. Ann Plast Surg 2022;88(2):S134–7.
49. Shu F, Liu H, Louet al. X. Analysis of the predictors of hypertrophic scarring pain and neuropathic pain after burn. Burns 2021;48(6):1425–34. https://doi.org/10.1016/j.burns.2021.08.007. Available at: Accessed June 20, 2022.
50. Klifto KM, Hultman CS, Dellon AL. Nerve Pain after Burn Injury: A Proposed Etiology-Based Classification. Plast Reconstr Surg 2021;635–44.
51. Tirado-Esteban A, Luis Seoane J, Domènech JS, et al. Sensory alteration patterns in burned patients. Burns 2019;46(8):1729–36. https://doi.org/10.1016/j.burns.2019.08.005. Available at: Accessed June 20, 2022.

Current Concepts in Surgical Management of Lymphedema

Rebecca Knackstedt, MD, PhD, Wei F. Chen, MD, FACS*

KEYWORDS

- Lymphedema • Lymphatic surgery • Lymphaticovenous bypass
- Vascularized lymph node transfer • Vascularized lymph vessel transfer
- Lymphatic surgery outcomes

KEY POINTS

- There is no formal consensus on what constitutes success or failure of complex decongestive therapy for lymphedema and when best to use surgical management.
- Recent evidence shows that early surgical intervention for lymphedema can delay, prevent, and even reverse lymphatic degeneration.
- The indications for various surgical interventions for lymphedema are being revisited and revised based on emerging research.

 Video content accompanies this article at http://www.pmr.theclinics.com.

INTRODUCTION

Although it has been estimated that approximately 200 million people worldwide and 3 to 5 million people in the United States suffer from lymphedema,[1–3] in reality, the true incidence of lymphedema is unknown. A diagnosis of lymphedema is often made purely based on clinical examination. However, variations in examination technique and the subjectivity associated with this approach have likely led to a large degree of under diagnosis. The successful treatment of lymphedema requires a multidisciplinary approach. The decision on whom to offer surgical interventions requires collaboration and input from all involved specialists and should address patients' expectations, invasiveness of procedures and disease severity.

Conflict of Interest: None.
Department of Plastic Surgery, Center for Lymphedema Research and Reconstruction, Cleveland Clinic, 2049 East 100th Street, A60, Cleveland, OH 44195, USA
* Corresponding author. Department of Plastic Surgery, Cleveland Clinic, 2049 East 100th Street, A60, Cleveland, OH 44195.
E-mail address: chenw6@ccf.org

Phys Med Rehabil Clin N Am 33 (2022) 885–899
https://doi.org/10.1016/j.pmr.2022.06.003
1047-9651/22/© 2022 Elsevier Inc. All rights reserved.

CLINICAL PRESENTATION AND WORKUP

The diagnosis of lymphedema is typically made clinically, although the severity of swelling does not always correlate with degree of lymphatic damage and disease. Lymphedema progresses in a predictable fashion, beginning with fluid-predominant disease that transitions to solid-predominant disease. Spontaneous infections are then able to occur, which leads to fibrosis. Fibrosis initially begins deep and progresses to involve superficial tissues and the skin. An extremity affected by lymphedema can manifest different stages of lymphedema, typically with worse disease distally due to gravity and extremity dependency.

A common cutoff for a diagnosis of lymphedema on clinical examination is a 2-cm difference between the affected and normal extremity.[4] However, this may be a normal variant that, without a suspicion for lymphedema, would have never been recognized. The stemmer sign is typically cited as differentiating between fluid and solid-predominant lymphedema.[5] Once again, this is a very subjective measurement. Additionally, studies have demonstrated that histologic changes can be observed in lymphatic vessels even before the onset of lymphedema.[6] Thus, for these patients, the disease process began well before a clinical diagnosis was made.

IMAGING

Lymphedema is characterized by lymphatic vessel ectasia and valve dysfunction, which allows lymphatic fluid to reflux into the interstitial space. Lymphatic fluid stasis leads to a localized inflammatory process, which causes extracellular matrix remodeling, adipose tissue differentiation, and progressive fibrosis/sclerosis with obliteration of the lymphatic vessel lumen.[6–9] These changes can be observed and tracked on imaging, the best objective means to diagnosis and monitor lymphedema.

Lymphoscintigraphy is considered by most to be the first-line imaging modality to analyze lymphedema. It allows for qualitative and quantitative analysis and is 96% to 100% sensitive and specific in the diagnosis of lymphedema.[10–14] However, reliable studies of lymphoscintigraphy staging systems[15–18] are lacking, and variations between injection and imaging protocols can make staging difficult.[19] Additionally, lymphoscintigraphy has poor spatial resolution and obligatory radiation exposure.

Indocyanine green (ICG) lymphography has higher sensitivity and specificity for diagnosing lymphedema compared with lymphoscintigraphy.[20] ICG can be injected peripherally, and it is taken up by the lymphatic system for analysis of the lymphatic vessels and flow.[21–23] This allows for real-time imaging, which permits calculation of flow velocity and analysis of the pump function. It delivers detailed anatomic information as opposed to the fuzzy qualitative imaging observed with lymphoscintography. The observed patterns can then be correlated with disease severity.[22,24] Drawbacks of ICG include an observation depth of only 2 cm, preventing analysis of deeper lymphatic systems. Although the optimal tool for analyzing the lymphatic system is yet to be determined, for now, ICG is currently the most useful. In the senior author's practice, ICG lymphography has largely replaced lymphoscintigraphy as the imaging modality of choice for diagnosis, preoperative planning, and postoperative monitoring.[25,26] The senior author does not perform any surgical intervention before obtaining imaging, which guides the decision of surgical approach.

STAGING

The original models of lymphedema staging focused on subjective findings without addressing onset or treatment planning.[27] However, these staging systems were created when little was understood about lymphedema and imaging options were limited. Since then, imaging modalities have been suggested as adjuncts to clarify staging.[15,19,24,28–32] These staging systems typically use ICG lymphography to evaluate lymphatic transport, presence of functional lymphatic vessels, and pattern and distribution of dermal backflow.[22,24,32–34] There are now different staging systems for upper and lower extremity lymphedema.[22,23] In the senior author's opinion, clinical staging systems are not crucial for surgical planning. What actually matters is the degree of lymphatic injury, which does not always agree with clinical staging and should be what guides surgical approach.

CONSERVATIVE THERAPY

Lymphedema in its early forms can be treated with complex decongestive therapy (CDT). CDT focuses on manual lymphatic drainage (MLD) through bandaging, skin and nail care, and exercise.[35–38] After lymph volume reduction is achieved and there is minimal or no pitting edema, maintenance therapy is performed.[39,40] Because CDT manages and does not cure lymphedema, it requires lifelong strict patient adherence. CDT is an option for patients who do not desire surgical intervention, are not surgical candidates, or have well-controlled, mild lymphedema. There are many unanswered questions surrounding CDT that modern technologies are allowing research to currently investigate. For example, the optimal pressure during MLD is not agreed on and is an active area of research.

There is no formal consensus on what constitutes success or failure of CDT. Because failure of CDT is considered by many surgeons to be the endpoint to prompt surgery, this warrants discussion. Success could be determined based on symptom relief, functional improvement, volume reduction, or patient expectations. It is our hope that therapists will continue to analyze their results and determine proper treatment endpoints to help guide the overall treatment algorithm. Although conservative therapy and surgery can both be beneficial for patients, there is not a consensus of timing for interventions and if they should be performed simultaneous or sequential.

SURGICAL TREATMENT OPTIONS

Recent evidence show that early surgical intervention for lymphedema can delay, prevent, and even reverse lymphatic degeneration.[41,42] Thus, although surgery has typically been considered a second-line intervention after conservative therapy failed, recent evidence argue for earlier surgery for certain patients. Surgical results are often more favorable the earlier in the disease course that they are performed. Lymphedema surgery can be categorized broadly into physiologic or debulking procedures.[43]

Debulking procedures have typically been considered optimal for patients with solid-predominant lymphedema. This can be demonstrated on physical examination and confirmed with imaging, such as an MRI. Debulking procedures remove diseased tissue and include liposuction[44–46] and the rarely performed Charles procedure.[47,48] The choice of liposuction or Charles procedure depends on the severity of the subcutaneous fibrosis.

Our group performs liposuction with simultaneous contouring skin reduction, the "flying squirrel" technique (**Fig. 1**, Video 1).[46,49] Liposuction cannot address severe subcutaneous tissue fibrosis. Thus, for these patients, direct excision is required.[47,48] In the senior author's experience, some patients that seem eligible for liposuction on physical examination may actually have very fibrotic tissue that can only be appreciated in the operating room, requiring a last-minute change of surgical approach to an excision. In these excision procedures, the skin is preserved when possible, and

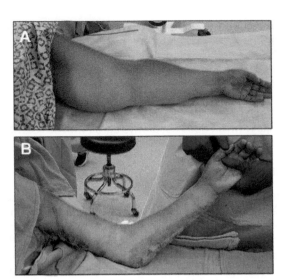

Fig. 1. Results that can be achieved with "flying squirrel" liposuction with skin excision. (*A*) Preoperative and (*B*) immediate postoperative.

radical resection with perforator preservation can be performed if the skin is not too fibrotic.[48]

The Charles procedure is not without risk because it can lead to fluid shifts, blood loss, and wound infections. However, with proper planning and attention to details, it can be a life-changing intervention for patients.[50]

Patients who undergo debulking procedures may still be candidates for secondary reconstructive procedures. However, the most effective sequence when multiple surgical procedures are to be used is yet to be determined.

Physiologic procedures rely on supermicrosurgery to restore or augment lymphatic drainage and include lymphaticovenular anastomosis (LVA)/bypass,[51–54] vascularized lymph node transfer (VLNT),[55–62] vascularized lymph vessel transfer (VLVT),[63,64] and lymph node to vein anastomosis (LNVA).[65] These procedures have historically been indicated for fluid predominant lymphedema.[66–70]

Modern lymphatic reconstruction was founded in the 1990s by Dr Hung-Chi Chen's creation of lymph node transfer.[55,71–76] Koshima then introduced supermicrosurgery with microvascular anastomosis for vessels of 0.3 to 0.8 mm.[77] This allowed for the creation of LVA to bypass obstructed lymphatic pathways (**Fig. 2**)[51,53,54] Vascularized lymph node transplant, the transferring healthy lymph nodes from one part of the body to a region that is impacted by lymphedema, was introduced by Koshima in 2016.[63] Koshima then furthered the field by introducing VLVT, which transfers lymphatic vessels without nodes, in 2016.[63] With ultrathin supermicrosurgical tissue transfer technique, Chen created 2 additional VLVT techniques, allowing safe transfers of axillary and groin lymph vessels (**Fig. 3**, groin VLVT; Video 2).[78]

The ability of the surgeon to identify patent and contractile lymphatic channels become more difficult as lymphedema becomes chronic.[79] For therapeutic LVA, in our experience, the more drainage pathways that can be created, the better the outcome, until a point of diminishing return.[68,80,81] For patients with early-stage lymphedema and high-quality "linear" patterns on ICG lymphography, it is anticipated that symptoms will improve soon after surgery. For patients with "diffuse" pattern on ICG lymphography, but imaging confirmed fluid-predominant disease, it is also

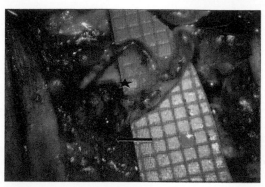

Fig. 2. Example LVA with 1 side-to-end (*star*) and 2 end-to-end (*arrow*) anastomoses.

expected that the symptoms will improve shortly after surgery.[68,82–86] Because surgery allows for the release of lymphatic pressure in these patients, the nonsclerotic lymphatic vessels can return to their functional state and allow for continual improvement.[80] For patients with fluid-predominant lymphedema, the limb volume typically changes significantly in the first 3 to 6 months and can improve up to 12 months or longer.[51,53,87] For patients with stage 3 and 4 lymphedema, the volume change is typically less significant due to the solid component but volume reduction is still observed.[80] A meta-analysis identified 22 studies that reported on outcomes with therapeutic LVA. Eighty-nine percent of patients reported subjective improvement, 88% experienced a quantitative improvement, and 56% of patients were able to discontinue compression therapy.[70]

Examples of commonly used VLNT include the groin,[56,62] supraclavicular,[59,88–90] submental[60] (**Fig. 4**), lateral thoracic,[91–94] omental,[95,96] and the jejunal mesenteric flaps.[97,98] Traditionally, the superficial circumflex iliac artery-based groin flap has served as the workhorse of VLNT, due to its reliable anatomy, abundant lymph nodes, and well-hidden scar.[56,99–101] In patients undergoing postmastectomy breast reconstruction, VLNT may be performed through a chimeric deep inferior epigastric artery perforator flap with groin vascularized lymph node flap.[57,100–102] To have a successful VLNT outcome, the identification of the functional lymph node becomes crucial.[65] Thus, in these operations, the surgical plan is sometimes altered to an LVA if functional nodes cannot be identified. Although VLNT is a relatively safe procedure, the risk of donor site lymphedema has not been eliminated.[94,103–107]

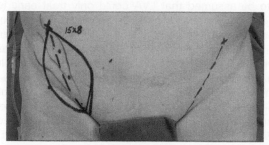

Fig. 3. Preoperative markings for groin-based thing superficial circumflex perforator VLVT flap. Black outline marks boundaries of flap, green marks vessels, and red marks lymph vessel location.

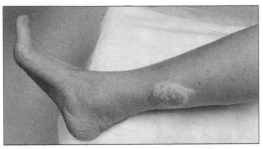

Fig. 4. Example of contour that can be achieved with submental lymph node free flap for lower extremity lymphedema.

The mechanism of VLNT is not understood but 2 mechanisms have been proposed.[55,108–114] One is through lymphangiogenesis with new afferent and efferent lymphatic collateral pathways connecting the transplanted lymph nodes with lymphatic vessels in the recipient site. This is thought to be mediated by lymphangiogenic growth factor secretion, including vascular endothelial growth factor-C (VEGF-C), from the transplanted lymph nodes.[108,115,116] The other is through neolymphangiogenesis in which new lymphaticovenous drainage pathways are created within the transplanted lymph nodes driven by perfusion gradients.[55,111,112,114] Similar to VLNT, the mechanism of VLVT is yet to be fully elucidated. It has been proposed that VLVT functions through the peristaltic, pumping actions of healthy lymphatic vessels that help transport accumulated lymph fluid into the venous system.[63,112] VLNT may also work through lymphangiogenesis.[108,112,117]

The recently revitalized LNVA by Hong offers another approach to lymphedema treatment.[65] The first experimental reports of LNVA were performed on a dog mesenteric lymph node being transected and the distal node with afferent lymphatic channels implanted into the inferior vena cava. Although this showed encouraging results,[118] early clinical results were not constant.[118–120] A recent report of 160 unilateral stages II and III lower extremity lymphedema compared outcomes between LNVA + LVA group to LVA only. The LNVA + LVA group showed significantly better results in circumference reduction, body weight reduction, and extracellular fluid reduction of the affected limb as compared with the LVA only group.[65] Future research is required to determine the role of this surgical procedure to treat lymphedema.

Conventional teaching has been to treat early fluid-predominant lymphedema with LVA, late fluid-predominant lymphedema with VLNT or VLVT and solid disease with liposuction or the Charles procedure. However, this dogma has undergone recent scrutiny. It used to be assumed that LVA could only treat early lymphedema and that the absence of "linear" patterns on ICG lymphography and/or the presence of venous insufficiency contraindicated its use.[59,121–123] However, recent reports have found that LVA can be successful even in moderate-to-severe disease.[124] With these LVA successes, the indications for LVA versus VLNT or VLVT are blurring.

Because physiologic procedures do not treat fat deposits, there are still indications for liposuction, with or without skin excision. Debulking and physiologic procedures can also be combined in the same or different anatomic regions. For example, a patient with fatty tissue in the upper arm may benefit from liposuction with skin removal proximally and LVA or VLNT or VLVT distally. The precise timing of these sequential procedures has yet to be determined. In our practice, if liposuction and a physiologic procedure are combined in the same anatomic region, they are performed 6 months apart to allow for scar relaxation after liposuction. Interestingly, unpublished results from the senior author demonstrate that the liposuction, with or without skin excision, results in improved lymph flow, even without a concomitant physiologic procedure. Thus, patients with fluid and fat predominant disease who undergo liposuction may not require a physiologic procedure. The mechanism of this success is not fully elucidated.

Controversy also surrounds the management of primary lymphedema, which is actually quite common. Primary lymphedema is not always hereditary but can often be sporadic in nature. Clinicians must be aware of this disease state and its prevalence because its treatment is different from that of secondary lymphedema. Many surgeons recommend VLNT over LVA for primary lymphedema due to theoretic concerns that the abnormal structure and function of lymphatics in these patients may decrease the efficacy of LVA.[42,125,126] However, in our experience, it is not uncommon for patients with primary lymphedema to exhibit global lymphatic dysfunction, as evidenced on ICG lymphography. This would preclude any flap transfer procedure due to an elevated risk of iatrogenic donor-site lymphedema, leaving LVA as a safer alternative.[23,127]

TRACKING OF OUTCOMES/EXPECTED OUTCOMES

After surgical intervention, patient outcomes can be measured subjectively and objectively with self-assessment, bioimpedance spectroscopy,[82] ICG lymphography,[68,80,128] limb circumference measurements, water displacement, tissue tonometry, perometer, and contrast-enhanced magnetic resonance lymphangiography. We recommend that postoperative outcome monitoring should be multimodal with a comprehensive clinical assessment.[80] It is our practice to perform ICG lymphangiography 3 months postoperatively to visualize and assess flow.[128] This is repeated at 6 and 12 months and then yearly.[128]

With surgical advances, lymphedema is more treatable than ever before, and many suboptimal results presented in the literature are likely due to inexperience of surgeons. Lymphedema surgery is meticulous and associated with a wide learning curve. However, when performed by an experienced surgeon, results can be extremely favorable.

SUMMARY

Optimal lymphedema management requires collaboration between multiple medical and surgical disciplines. Emerging research is elucidating the pathophysiology of lymphedema and mechanism of surgical improvement. Future research will help clarify when to use surgical interventions and which procedures are optimal for a given patient. These unanswered questions will be best addressed through well-done, prospective studies and multi-institutional collaboration.

CLINICS CARE POINTS

- Lymphedema is not, and should not be, a clinical diagnosis. The diagnosis needs to be definitive and therefore rquires confirmatory imaging study.

- Effective lymphedema treatments, both surgical and non-surgical, exist today. The common misconception held by patients that "there is no effective treatment for lymphedema" should be corrected. The patients should be encouraged to seek out appropriate specialists for lymphedema management.

- Lymphedema surgery can favorably and fundamentally affect disease pathophysiology, but at the cost of being invasive.

- When appropriate surgical procedure is performed in properly selected patients by experienced lymphedema micro- and supermicro-surgeon, the outcome is frequently highly favorable.
- Further research are needed in delineating surgical candidacy, deciding which procedure to perform, the timing of surgical intervention, and long-term outcomes.

FINANCIAL DISCLOSURE AND PRODUCTS PAGE

None of the authors has a financial interest in any of the products, devices, or drugs mentioned in this article.

SUPPLEMENTARY DATA

Supplementary data related to this article can be found online at https://doi.org/10.1016/j.pmr.2022.06.003.

REFERENCES

1. Cemal Y, Pusic A, Mehrara BJ. Preventative measures for lymphedema: separating fact from fiction. J Am Coll Surg 2011;213(4):543–51.
2. Rockson SG, Rivera KK. Estimating the population burden of lymphedema. Ann N Y Acad Sci 2008;1131:147–54.
3. Rebegea L, Firescu D, Dumitru M, et al. The incidence and risk factors for occurrence of arm lymphedema after treatment of breast cancer. Chirurgia (Bucur) 2015;110(1):33–7.
4. Can AG, Eksioglu E, Bahtiyarca ZT, et al. Assessment of Risk Factors in Patients who presented to the Outpatient Clinic for Breast Cancer-Related Lymphedema. J Breast Health 2016;12(1):31–6.
5. Goss JA, Greene AK. Sensitivity and Specificity of the Stemmer Sign for Lymphedema: A Clinical Lymphoscintigraphic Study. Plast Reconstr Surg Glob Open 2019;7(6):e2295.
6. Mihara M, Hara H, Hayashi Y, et al. Pathological steps of cancer-related lymphedema: histological changes in the collecting lymphatic vessels after lymphadenectomy. PloS one 2012;7(7):e41126.
7. Rutkowski JM, Swartz MA. A driving force for change: interstitial flow as a morphoregulator. Trends Cell Biology 2007;17(1):44–50.
8. Zampell JC, Yan A, Elhadad S, et al. CD4(+) cells regulate fibrosis and lymphangiogenesis in response to lymphatic fluid stasis. PloS one 2012;7(11):e49940.
9. Avraham T, Daluvoy S, Zampell J, et al. Blockade of transforming growth factor-beta1 accelerates lymphatic regeneration during wound repair. Am J Pathol 2010;177(6):3202–14.
10. Rossi M, Grassi R, Costa R, et al. Evaluation of the Upper Limb Lymphatic System: A Prospective Lymphoscintigraphic Study in Melanoma Patients and Healthy Controls. Plast Reconstr Surg 2016;138(6):1321–31.
11. Weissleder H, Weissleder R. Lymphedema: evaluation of qualitative and quantitative lymphoscintigraphy in 238 patients. Radiology 1988;167(3):729–35.
12. Vaqueiro M, Gloviczki P, Fisher J, et al. Lymphoscintigraphy in lymphedema: an aid to microsurgery. J Nucl Med 1986;27(7):1125–30.
13. Cambria RA, Gloviczki P, Naessens JM, et al. Noninvasive evaluation of the lymphatic system with lymphoscintigraphy: a prospective, semiquantitative analysis in 386 extremities. J Vasc Surg 1993;18(5):773–82.

14. Hassanein AH, Maclellan RA, Grant FD, et al. Diagnostic Accuracy of Lympho-scintigraphy for Lymphedema and Analysis of False-Negative Tests. Plast Re-constr Surg Glob Open 2017;5(7):e1396.

15. Szuba A, Shin WS, Strauss HW, et al. The third circulation: radionuclide lympho-scintigraphy in the evaluation of lymphedema. J Nucl Med 2003;44(1):43–57.

16. Pecking AP, Wartski M, Cluzan RV, et al. SPECT-CT fusion imaging radionuclide lymphoscintigraphy: potential for limb lymphedema assessment and sentinel node detection in breast cancer. Cancer Treat Res 2007;135:79–84.

17. Lee BB, Bergan JJ. New clinical and laboratory staging systems to improve management of chronic lymphedema. Lymphology 2005;38(3):122–9.

18. Maegawa J, Mikami T, Yamamoto Y, et al. Types of lymphoscintigraphy and in-dications for lymphaticovenous anastomosis. Microsurgery 2010;30(6):437–42.

19. Kramer EL. Lymphoscintigraphy: defining a clinical role. Lymphatic Res Biol 2004;2(1):32–7.

20. Mihara M, Hara H, Araki J, et al. Indocyanine green (ICG) lymphography is su-perior to lymphoscintigraphy for diagnostic imaging of early lymphedema of the upper limbs. PloS one 2012;7(6):e38182.

21. Yamamoto T, Narushima M, Doi K, et al. Characteristic indocyanine green lymphography findings in lower extremity lymphedema: the generation of a novel lymphedema severity staging system using dermal backflow patterns. Plast Reconstr Surg 2011;127(5):1979–86.

22. Yamamoto T, Yamamoto N, Doi K, et al. Indocyanine green-enhanced lymphog-raphy for upper extremity lymphedema: a novel severity staging system using dermal backflow patterns. Plast Reconstr Surg 2011;128(4):941–7.

23. Yamamoto T, Yoshimatsu H, Narushima M, et al. Indocyanine Green Lymphog-raphy Findings in Primary Leg Lymphedema. Eur J Vasc Endovasc Surg 2015; 49(1):95–102.

24. Yamamoto T, Matsuda N, Doi K, et al. The earliest finding of indocyanine green lymphography in asymptomatic limbs of lower extremity lymphedema patients secondary to cancer treatment: the modified dermal backflow stage and concept of subclinical lymphedema. Plast Reconstr Surg 2011;128(4): 314e–21e.

25. Yamamoto T, Iida T, Matsuda N, et al. Indocyanine green (ICG)-enhanced lymphography for evaluation of facial lymphoedema. J Plast Reconstr Aesthet Surg 2011;64(11):1541–4.

26. Mihara M, Hara H, Narushima M, et al. Indocyanine green lymphography is su-perior to lymphoscintigraphy in imaging diagnosis of secondary lymphedema of the lower limbs. J Vasc Surg Venous Lymphat Disord 2013;1(2):194–201.

27. International Society of L. The diagnosis and treatment of peripheral lymphe-dema: 2013 Consensus Document of the International Society of Lymphology. Lymphology 2013;46(1):1–11.

28. Vaughan BF. CT of swollen legs. Clin Radiol 1990;41(1):24–30.

29. Dimakakos PB, Stefanopoulos T, Antoniades P, et al. MRI and ultrasonographic findings in the investigation of lymphedema and lipedema. Int Surg 1997;82(4): 411–6.

30. Arrive L, Azizi L, Lewin M, et al. MR lymphography of abdominal and retroper-itoneal lymphatic vessels. AJR Am J Roentgenol 2007;189(5):1051–8.

31. Neligan PC, Kung TA, Maki JH. MR lymphangiography in the treatment of lym-phedema. J Surg Oncol 2017;115(1):18–22.

32. Chang DW, Suami H, Skoracki R. A prospective analysis of 100 consecutive lymphovenous bypass cases for treatment of extremity lymphedema. Plast Reconstr Surg 2013;132(5):1305–14.

33. Narushima M, Yamamoto T, Ogata F, et al. Indocyanine Green Lymphography Findings in Limb Lymphedema. J Reconstr Microsurg 2016;32(1):72–9.

34. Hara H, Mihara M, Seki Y, et al. Comparison of indocyanine green lymphographic findings with the conditions of collecting lymphatic vessels of limbs in patients with lymphedema. Plast Reconstr Surg 2013;132(6):1612–8.

35. Ko DS, Lerner R, Klose G, et al. Effective treatment of lymphedema of the extremities. Arch Surg 1998;133(4):452–8.

36. Szuba A, Cooke JP, Yousuf S, et al. Decongestive lymphatic therapy for patients with cancer-related or primary lymphedema. Am J Med 2000;109(4):296–300.

37. Vignes S, Porcher R, Champagne A, et al. Predictive factors of response to intensive decongestive physiotherapy in upper limb lymphedema after breast cancer treatment: a cohort study. Breast Cancer Res Treat 2006;98(1):1–6.

38. Chang DW, Masia J, Garza R 3rd, et al. Lymphedema: Surgical and Medical Therapy. Plast Reconstr Surg 2016;138(3 Suppl):209S–18S.

39. Schaverien MV, Moeller JA, Cleveland SD. Nonoperative Treatment of Lymphedema. Semin Plast Surg 2018;32(1):17–21.

40. Rodrick JR, Poage E, Wanchai A, et al. Complementary, alternative, and other noncomplete decongestive therapy treatment methods in the management of lymphedema: a systematic search and review. PM R 2014;6(3):250–74 [quiz: 274].

41. Torrisi JS, Joseph WJ, Ghanta S, et al. Lymphaticovenous bypass decreases pathologic skin changes in upper extremity breast cancer-related lymphedema. Lymphat Res Biol 2015;13(1):46–53.

42. Garza RM, Chang DW. Lymphovenous bypass for the treatment of lymphedema. J Surg Oncol 2018;118(5):743–9.

43. Garza R 3rd, Skoracki R, Hock K, et al. A comprehensive overview on the surgical management of secondary lymphedema of the upper and lower extremities related to prior oncologic therapies. BMC Cancer 2017;17(1):468.

44. Hoffner M, Ohlin K, Svensson B, et al. Liposuction Gives Complete Reduction of Arm Lymphedema following Breast Cancer Treatment-A 5-year Prospective Study in 105 Patients without Recurrence. Plast Reconstr Surg Glob Open 2018;6(8):e1912.

45. Boyages J, Kastanias K, Koelmeyer LA, et al. Liposuction for Advanced Lymphedema: A Multidisciplinary Approach for Complete Reduction of Arm and Leg Swelling. Ann Surg Oncol 2015;22(Suppl 3):S1263–70.

46. PJ Hawkes JD, Bowen M, Chen Wi F. Suction Assisted Lipectomy With Immediate Limb Contouring for Advanced, Solid-Predominant Lymphedema. Ann Plast Surg 2018;80(4):1.

47. Chalres RH. The surgical technique and operative treatment of elephantiasis of the generative organs based on a series of 140 consecutive successful cases. Indian Med Gaz 1901;36:16.

48. Sapountzis S, Ciudad P, Lim SY, et al. Modified Charles procedure and lymph node flap transfer for advanced lower extremity lymphedema. Microsurgery 2014;34(6):439–47.

49. Schaverien MV, Munnoch DA, Brorson H. Liposuction Treatment of Lymphedema. Semin Plast Surg 2018;32(1):42–7.

50. Hassan K, Chang DW. The Charles Procedure as Part of the Modern Armamentarium Against Lymphedema. Ann Plast Surg 2020;85(6):e37–43.

51. Koshima I, Inagawa K, Etoh K, et al. [Supramicrosurgical lymphaticovenular anastomosis for the treatment of lymphedema in the extremities]. Nihon Geka Gakkai Zasshi 1999;100(9):551-6.

52. Giacalone G, Yamamoto T, Hayashi A, et al. Lymphatic supermicrosurgery for the treatment of recurrent lymphocele and severe lymphorrhea. Microsurgery 2019;39(4):326-31.

53. Koshima I, Inagawa K, Urushibara K, et al. Supermicrosurgical lymphaticovenular anastomosis for the treatment of lymphedema in the upper extremities. J Reconstr Microsurg 2000;16(6):437-42.

54. Koshima I, Nanba Y, Tsutsui T, et al. Long-term follow-up after lymphaticovenular anastomosis for lymphedema in the leg. J Reconstr Microsurg 2003;19(4):209-15.

55. Chen HC, O'Brien BM, Rogers IW, et al. Lymph node transfer for the treatment of obstructive lymphoedema in the canine model. Br J Plast Surg 1990;43(5):578-86.

56. Lin CH, Ali R, Chen SC, et al. Vascularized groin lymph node transfer using the wrist as a recipient site for management of postmastectomy upper extremity lymphedema. Plast Reconstr Surg 2009;123(4):1265-75.

57. Becker C, Assouad J, Riquet M, et al. Postmastectomy lymphedema: long-term results following microsurgical lymph node transplantation. Ann Surg 2006;243(3):313-5.

58. Batista BN, Germain M, Faria JC, et al. Lymph node flap transfer for patients with secondary lower limb lymphedema. Microsurgery 2017;37(1):29-33.

59. Mardonado AA, Chen R, Chang DW. The use of supraclavicular free flap with vascularized lymph node transfer for treatment of lymphedema: A prospective study of 100 consecutive cases. J Surg Oncol 2017;115(1):68-71.

60. Cheng MH, Huang JJ, Nguyen DH, et al. A novel approach to the treatment of lower extremity lymphedema by transferring a vascularized submental lymph node flap to the ankle. Gynecol Oncol 2012;126(1):93-8.

61. Gould DJ, Mehrara BJ, Neligan P, et al. Lymph node transplantation for the treatment of lymphedema. J Surg Oncol 2018;118(5):736-42.

62. Cheng MH, Chen SC, Henry SL, et al. Vascularized groin lymph node flap transfer for postmastectomy upper limb lymphedema: flap anatomy, recipient sites, and outcomes. Plast Reconstr Surg 2013;131(6):1286-98.

63. Koshima I, Narushima M, Mihara M, et al. Lymphadiposal Flaps and Lymphaticovenular Anastomoses for Severe Leg Edema: Functional Reconstruction for Lymph Drainage System. J Reconstr Microsurg 2016;32(1):50-5.

64. Chen WF, Bowen M, McNurlen M, et al. Vascularized Lymph Vessel Transfer with Supermicrosurgical Ultra-Thin Superficial Circumflex Iliac Artery Flap for Treatment of Advanced Lymphedema not Treatable with Supermicrosurgical Lymphaticovenular Anastomosis. Ann Plast Surg 2018;80(supp 3):1.

65. Pak CS, Suh HP, Kwon JG, et al. Lymph Node to Vein Anastomosis (LNVA) for lower extremity lymphedema. J Plast Reconstr Aesthet Surg 2021;74(9):2059-67.

66. Brorson H. Liposuction in Lymphedema Treatment. J Reconstr microsurg 2016;32(1):56-65.

67. Brorson H, Svensson H. Liposuction combined with controlled compression therapy reduces arm lymphedema more effectively than controlled compression therapy alone. Plast Reconstr Surg 1998;102(4):1058-67 [discussion: 1068].

68. Chen WF. How to Get Started Performing Supermicrosurgical Lymphaticovenular Anastomosis to Treat Lymphedema. Ann Plast Surg 2018;81(6S Suppl 1): S15–20.

69. Pappalardo M, Patel K, Cheng MH. Vascularized lymph node transfer for treatment of extremity lymphedema: An overview of current controversies regarding donor sites, recipient sites and outcomes. J Surg Oncol 2018;117(7):1420–31.

70. Basta MN, Gao LL, Wu LC. Operative treatment of peripheral lymphedema: a systematic meta-analysis of the efficacy and safety of lymphovenous microsurgery and tissue transplantation. Plast Reconstr Surg 2014;133(4):905–13.

71. Salgado CJ, Sassu P, Gharb BB, et al. Radical reduction of upper extremity lymphedema with preservation of perforators. Ann Plast Surg 2009;63(3):302–6.

72. Karri V, Yang MC, Lee IJ, et al. Optimizing outcome of charles procedure for chronic lower extremity lymphoedema. Ann Plast Surg 2011;66(4):393–402.

73. Yeo MS, Lim SY, Kiranantawat K, et al. A comparison of vascularized cervical lymph node transfer with and without modified Charles' procedure for the treatment of lower limb lymphedema. Plast Reconstr Surg 2014;134(1):171e–2e.

74. Visconti G, Brunelli C, Mule A, et al. Septum-based cervical lymph-node free flap in rat: a new model. J Surg Res 2016;201(1):1–12.

75. Visconti G, Constantinescu T, Chen PY, et al. The Venous Lymph Node Flap: Concepts, Experimental Evidence, and Potential Clinical Implications. J Reconstr Microsurg 2016;32(8):625–31.

76. Ciudad P, Mouchammed A, Manrique OJ, et al. Comparison of long-term clinical outcomes among different vascularized lymph node transfers: 6-year experience of a single center's approach to the treatment of lymphedema. J Surg Oncol 2018;117(6):1346–7.

77. Masia J, Olivares L, Koshima I, et al. Barcelona consensus on supermicrosurgery. J Reconstr Microsurg 2014;30(1):53–8.

78. Chen WM M, Ding J, Bowen M. Vascularized Lymph Vessel Transfer for Extremity Lymphedema - Is Transfer of Lymph Node Still Necessary. Int Microsurgery J 2019;3.

79. Silva AK, Chang DW. Vascularized lymph node transfer and lymphovenous bypass: Novel treatment strategies for symptomatic lymphedema. J Surg Oncol 2016;113(8):932–9.

80. Chen WF, Bowen M, Ding J. Lessons learned after 100 cases supermicrosurgical lymphaticovenular anastomosis - a single surgeons' experience. Ann Plast Surg 2018;80(spp 3):1.

81. Chen WF, Yamamoto T, Fisher M, et al. The "Octopus" Lymphaticovenular Anastomosis: Evolving Beyond the Standard Supermicrosurgical Technique. J Reconstr Microsurg 2015;31(6):450–7.

82. Qin ES, Bowen MJ, Chen WF. Diagnostic accuracy of bioimpedance spectroscopy in patients with lymphedema: A retrospective cohort analysis. J Plast Reconstr Aesthet Surg 2018;71(7):1041–50.

83. Qin ES, Bowen MJ, James SL, et al. Multi-segment bioimpedance can assess patients with bilateral lymphedema. J Plast Reconstr Aesthet Surg 2020;73(2): 328–36.

84. Sen Y, Qian Y, Koelmeyer L, et al. Breast Cancer-Related Lymphedema: Differentiating Fat from Fluid Using Magnetic Resonance Imaging Segmentation. Lymphat Res Biol 2018;16(1):20–7.

85. Wang L, Wu X, Wu M, et al. Edema Areas of Calves Measured with Magnetic Resonance Imaging as a Novel Indicator for Early Staging of Lower Extremity Lymphedema. Lymphat Res Biol 2018;16(3):240–7.

86. Trinh L, Peterson P, Brorson H, et al. Assessment of Subfascial Muscle/Water and Fat Accumulation in Lymphedema Patients Using Magnetic Resonance Imaging. Lymphat Res Biol 2019;17(3):340–6.

87. Huang GK, Hu RQ, Liu ZZ, et al. Microlymphaticovenous anastomosis in the treatment of lower limb obstructive lymphedema: analysis of 91 cases. Plast Reconstr Surg 1985;76(5):671–85.

88. Akita S, Nakamura R, Yamamoto N, et al. Early Detection of Lymphatic Disorder and Treatment for Lymphedema following Breast Cancer. Plast Reconstr Surg 2016;138(2):192e–202e.

89. Sapountzis S, Singhal D, Rashid A, et al. Lymph node flap based on the right transverse cervical artery as a donor site for lymph node transfer. Ann Plast Surg 2014;73(4):398–401.

90. Steinbacher J, Tinhofer IE, Meng S, et al. The surgical anatomy of the supraclavicular lymph node flap: A basis for the free vascularized lymph node transfer. J Surg Oncol 2017;115(1):60–2.

91. Barreiro GC, Baptista RR, Kasai KE, et al. Lymph fasciocutaneous lateral thoracic artery flap: anatomical study and clinical use. J Reconstr Microsurg 2014;30(6):389–96.

92. Tinhofer IE, Meng S, Steinbacher J, et al. The surgical anatomy of the vascularized lateral thoracic artery lymph node flap-A cadaver study. J Surg Oncol 2017; 116(8):1062–8.

93. Smith ML, Molina BJ, Dayan E, et al. Heterotopic vascularized lymph node transfer to the medial calf without a skin paddle for restoration of lymphatic function: Proof of concept. J Surg Oncol 2017;115(1):90–5.

94. Dayan JH, Dayan E, Smith ML. Reverse lymphatic mapping: a new technique for maximizing safety in vascularized lymph node transfer. Plast Reconstr Surg 2015;135(1):277–85.

95. Ciudad P, Agko M, Perez Coca JJ, et al. Comparison of long-term clinical outcomes among different vascularized lymph node transfers: 6-year experience of a single center's approach to the treatment of lymphedema. J Surg Oncol 2017;116(6):671–82.

96. Nguyen AT, Suami H, Hanasono MM, et al. Long-term outcomes of the minimally invasive free vascularized omental lymphatic flap for the treatment of lymphedema. J Surg Oncol 2017;115(1):84–9.

97. Coriddi M, Skoracki R, Eiferman D. Vascularized jejunal mesenteric lymph node transfer for treatment of extremity lymphedema. Microsurgery 2017;37(2): 177–8.

98. Schaverien MV, Hofstetter WL, Selber JC. Vascularized Jejunal Mesenteric Lymph Node Transfer for Lymphedema: A Novel Approach. Plast Reconstr Surg 2018;141(3):468e–9e.

99. Allen RJ Jr, Cheng MH. Lymphedema surgery: Patient selection and an overview of surgical techniques. J Surg Oncol 2016;113(8):923–31.

100. Saaristo AM, Niemi TS, Viitanen TP, et al. Microvascular breast reconstruction and lymph node transfer for postmastectomy lymphedema patients. Ann Surg 2012;255(3):468–73.

101. Nguyen AT, Chang EI, Suami H, et al. An algorithmic approach to simultaneous vascularized lymph node transfer with microvascular breast reconstruction. Ann Surg Oncol 2015;22(9):2919–24.

102. Akita S, Tokumoto H, Yamaji Y, et al. Contribution of Simultaneous Breast Reconstruction by Deep Inferior Epigastric Artery Perforator Flap to the Efficacy of

Vascularized Lymph Node Transfer in Patients with Breast Cancer-Related Lymphedema. J Reconstr Microsurg 2017;33(8):571–8.

103. Azuma S, Yamamoto T, Koshima I. Donor-site lymphatic function after microvascular lymph node transfer should be followed using indocyanine green lymphography. Plast Reconstr Surg 2013;131(3):443e–4e.

104. Vignes S, Blanchard M, Yannoutsos A, et al. Complications of autologous lymph-node transplantation for limb lymphoedema. Eur J Vasc Endovasc Surg 2013; 45(5):516–20.

105. Pons G, Masia J, Loschi P, et al. A case of donor-site lymphoedema after lymph node-superficial circumflex iliac artery perforator flap transfer. J Plast Reconstr Aesthet Surg 2014;67(1):119–23.

106. Goh TL, Park SW, Cho JY, et al. The search for the ideal thin skin flap: superficial circumflex iliac artery perforator flap–a review of 210 cases. Plast Reconstr Surg 2015;135(2):592–601.

107. Coriddi M, Wee C, Meyerson J, et al. Vascularized Jejunal Mesenteric Lymph Node Transfer: A Novel Surgical Treatment for Extremity Lymphedema. J Am Coll Surg 2017;225(5):650–7.

108. Shesol BF, Nakashima R, Alavi A, et al. Successful lymph node transplantation in rats, with restoration of lymphatic function. Plast Reconstr Surg 1979;63(6): 817–23.

109. Patel KM, Lin CY, Cheng MH. From theory to evidence: long-term evaluation of the mechanism of action and flap integration of distal vascularized lymph node transfers. J Reconstr Microsurg 2015;31(1):26–30.

110. Suami H, Scaglioni MF, Dixon KA, et al. Interaction between vascularized lymph node transfer and recipient lymphatics after lymph node dissection-a pilot study in a canine model. J Surg Res 2016;204(2):418–27.

111. Ito R, Zelken J, Yang CY, et al. Proposed pathway and mechanism of vascularized lymph node flaps. Gynecol Oncol 2016;141(1):182–8.

112. Cheng MH, Huang JJ, Wu CW, et al. The mechanism of vascularized lymph node transfer for lymphedema: natural lymphaticovenous drainage. Plast Reconstr Surg 2014;133(2):192e–8e.

113. Yan A, Avraham T, Zampell JC, et al. Mechanisms of lymphatic regeneration after tissue transfer. PloS one 2011;6(2):e17201.

114. Aschen SZ, Farias-Eisner G, Cuzzone DA, et al. Lymph node transplantation results in spontaneous lymphatic reconnection and restoration of lymphatic flow. Plast Reconstr Surg 2014;133(2):301–10.

115. Viitanen TP, Visuri MT, Hartiala P, et al. Lymphatic vessel function and lymphatic growth factor secretion after microvascular lymph node transfer in lymphedema patients. Plast Reconstr Surg Glob open 2013;1(2):1–9.

116. Huang JJ, Gardenier JC, Hespe GE, et al. Lymph Node Transplantation Decreases Swelling and Restores Immune Responses in a Transgenic Model of Lymphedema. PloS one 2016;11(12):e0168259.

117. Can J, Cai R, Li S, et al. Experimental study of lymph node auto-transplantation in rats. Chin Med J 1998;111(3):239–41.

118. Calnan JS, Reis ND, Rivero OR, et al. The natural history of lymph node-to-vein anastomoses. Br J Plast Surg 1967;20(2):134–45.

119. Nielubowicz J, Olszewski W. Surgical lymphaticovenous shunts in patients with secondary lymphoedema. Br J Surg 1968;55(6):440–2.

120. Olszewski WL. The treatment of lymphedema of the extremities with microsurgical lympho-venous anastomoses. Int Angiol 1988;7(4):312–21.

121. Gallagher KK, Lopez M, Iles K, et al. Surgical Approach to Lymphedema Reduction. Curr Oncol Rep 2020;22(10):97.
122. Schaverien MV, Coroneos CJ. Surgical Treatment of Lymphedema. Plast Reconstr Surg 2019;144(3):738–58.
123. Masia J, Pons G, Nardulli ML. Combined Surgical Treatment in Breast Cancer-Related Lymphedema. J Reconstr Microsurg 2016;32(1):16–27.
124. Yang JC, Wu SC, Lin WC, et al. Supermicrosurgical Lymphaticovenous Anastomosis as Alternative Treatment Option for Moderate-to-Severe Lower Limb Lymphedema. J Am Coll Surg 2020;230(2):216–27.
125. Mihara M, Hara H, Furniss D, et al. Lymphaticovenular anastomosis to prevent cellulitis associated with lymphoedema. Br J Surg 2014;101(11):1391–6.
126. Drobot A, Bez M, Abu Shakra I, et al. Microsurgery for management of primary and secondary lymphedema. J Vasc Surg Venous Lymphat Disord 2021;9(1): 226–233 e221.
127. Giacalone G, Yamamoto T, Belva F, et al. The Application of Virtual Reality for Preoperative Planning of Lymphovenous Anastomosis in a Patient with a Complex Lymphatic Malformation. J Clin Med 2019;8(3):371.
128. Chen WF, Zhao H, Yamamoto T, et al. Indocyanine Green Lymphographic Evidence of Surgical Efficacy Following Microsurgical and Supermicrosurgical Lymphedema Reconstructions. J Reconstr Microsurg 2016;32(9):688–98.

Emerging Technologies in the Wound Management Field

George Marzloff, MD[a],*, Stephanie Ryder, MD[a],
Jennifer Hutton, MS, RN, CNS, CWCN, CRRN[a], Kaila Ott, MS, ATP[a],
Mallory Becker, RN, BSN, CWCN, CRRN[b], Scott Schubert, MD[a]

KEYWORDS

- Surfaces • Cushions • Pressure mapping • Imaging • Negative pressure
- Skin substitutes • Electrical stimulation • Ultrasound

KEY POINTS

- Technological advances are incorporated into all stages of wound care management.
- Modern mattresses and cushions are designed to distribute pressure to decrease the risk of pressure injury development or exacerbation, and the team uses pressure mapping technology for selecting the best surface for a patient.
- Image processing algorithms aid in three-dimensional wound monitoring, and multiple types of radiological studies are used to visualize affected tissue deep to the wound bed.
- Treating wounds often involves high tech therapies such as negative pressure with infusion, electrical stimulation, and ultrasound.

INTRODUCTION

One of the earliest artifacts that describes rudimentary wound care is a clay tablet that dates back to 2200 BC. It describes making plasters—usually a mixture of mud, plants, herbs, and oil, to place in the wound bed—followed by bandaging. Progress was limited for thousands of years until technological advances in surgery, antiseptic techniques, and antibiotics paved the way for the era of modern wound healing.[1] In this review, we discuss technologies for wounds that enhance (1) prevention through specialty mattresses and pressure mapping, (2) assessment using modern imaging, and (3) treatment with dressings and active therapies. We present these concepts in the context of managing patients with spinal cord injury (SCI), although the principles are applicable to other populations at risk for wounds.

---

[a] Rocky Mountain Regional VA Medical Center, 1700 N. Wheeling St (K1-11SC), Aurora, CO 80045, USA; [b] Elevance Health Companies, 220 Virginia Avenue, Indianapolis IN 46204, USA
* Corresponding author.
E-mail address: george.marzloff@va.gov

Phys Med Rehabil Clin N Am 33 (2022) 901–914
https://doi.org/10.1016/j.pmr.2022.06.005
1047-9651/22/Published by Elsevier Inc.

MATTRESSES

Although level I evidence for support surfaces is far from robust, it is the consensus that patients at high risk for pressure injury should be placed on specialty mattresses to redistribute pressure between patient and surface, reduce shear, and control moisture.[2] As nearly all patients with SCI will experience at least one pressure injury during their lifetimes, specialty surfaces should be used for both prevention and treatment of pressure injuries. Support surfaces for beds can be overlays applied over a standard mattress, replacement mattresses, or specialty beds, which are a mattress plus a bed frame.[3] Beyond the standard hospital mattress, there are low-tech static mattresses and overlays made of elastic material that can be used for the prevention and management of early stage wounds. For more complicated wounds, there are 3 high-tech categories of surfaces: alternating pressure, low-air-loss, and air-fluidized (**Table 1**).

High-level evidence to support one particular surface over another for both prevention and treatment of pressure injuries is limited,[4] and it is important to consider degree of immobility, ability to adhere to turns, current or prior pressure injuries, and body habitus when selecting a support surface.[5–7] A Cochrane Review found that foam static mattresses are better than standard hospital mattresses at reducing pressure injury incidence in high-risk patients, whereas alternating-pressure mattresses reduce cost and hospital length of stay compared with alternating-pressure overlays; other comparisons among support surfaces could not be definitively made due to small sample size and risk of bias in the studies.[2] A recent randomized controlled trial suggested benefits of alternating-pressure mattresses over high-specification foam mattresses but was limited by low incidence of pressure injury development during the study period.[8]

When strict bedrest is warranted and pressure on a complex pressure injury or a flap site is unavoidable, tissue compression between the support surface and bony prominences is exacerbated. In these situations, an adequate support surface would offload the patient to avoid excessive capillary pressure and maintain near-normal blood flow.[3,5] Historically, air-fluidized beds have been recommended because they are designed to simulate floating and promote adequate blood flow.[5] In our clinical practice, there are disadvantages to air-fluidized beds. First, many patients dislike the heat and noise. Second, bowel or bladder incontinence requires a complete change of the bed because it affects bead performance. Third, in our experience, new pressure injuries can occur on elbows, heels, or other body parts from the bumper surrounding the mattress without proper offloading. Small studies have questioned if other mattresses may be a cost-effective alternative in postflap scenarios.[8,9] Our center uses the reactive air pressure (marketed as fluid immersion simulation) beds most often, which monitors the support surface with microprocessors more than 100 times per second to provide constant adjustments according to patient positioning and generate an artificial fluid-immersion surface. These beds have shown a tendency to trap moisture under the patient due to less microclimate control, requiring frequent assessment and drying agents to prevent maceration.[10] Higher staff involvement is also needed for diligent turns and repositioning, particularly as patients may slide down due to the antishear surface.

To help in support surface selection, software has been developed to monitor the microclimate between the patient and support surface by evaluating temperature, moisture, and most commonly, pressure.[11,12] All of these measures suffer from lack of validated pressure values at which pressure injuries definitively heal.

Importantly, specialty support surfaces do not replace the need for other wound-mitigating strategies such as turns, padding to offload bony prominences, and

Table 1
Support surfaces—overlays, mattresses, and beds[2,4,5]

	Composition	Pros	Cons	Recommended Use
Standard mattress	Foam	• Cheapest • Readily available • No power needed	• No pressure distribution • No moisture control	• Patients at low risk for pressure injury
Low tech static mattresses/overlays: IsoFlex LAL	Materials (ie, foams, gels, air, water, beads, and so forth) mold around patient to distribute pressure	• Cheap • No power needed • Some pressure distribution • Transfers not affected	• No moisture control • No heat control • May have shearing	• Wound can still be offloaded by positioning on the mattress
High tech alternating pressure mattresses/overlays: Sizewise Pulsate	Air-filled sacs alternate inflation/deflation to vary pressure	• Intermittent pressure relief • Reduces shear	• Moderate cost • No moisture control • No heat control • Possible intermittent higher pressures • Requires electricity	• Unable to position off wound • Bottoming out or new pressure injury occurred on static surface
High tech low-air-loss beds/overlays: Völkner Turning System Dolphin Fluid Immersion Simulation	Warmed air flows through air sacs to vary pressure Reactive Air Pressure Mattress: Added microprocessors and software to constantly adjust to patient anatomy and movements, simulating fluid immersion	• Pressure relieving over a larger area • Reduces moisture • Reduces heat • May reduce shear • May also turn patient (Völkner) • May be reactive to movement (Dolphin®)	• Expensive • Can interfere with transfers, activities of daily living • May be noisy • Requires electricity • No microclimate control, can trap moisture	• Multiple pressure injuries that cannot be offloaded during turns • Large stage III or IV pressure injuries • Acute SCI after spine stabilization or postflap (Dolphin)
High tech air-fluidized beds: Clinitron Envella	Warmed air flows through small ceramic beads to vary pressure and simulate floating	• Pressure relieving over a larger area • Reduces moisture • Reduces shear	• Very expensive • Interferes with transfers, ADLs • High electricity needs • Hot • Loud • Risk of dehydration due to insensible losses	• Multiple pressure injuries that cannot be offloaded during turns • Large stage III or IV pressure injuries • Postflap surgery

maintaining a low degree of head-of-bed elevation. One study looking at 2 alternating air cell mattresses found that interface pressures greatly increased with head-of-bed elevation at 45°.[13] Another study found an 8% incidence of stage 1 and 2 pressure injuries in patients in a surgical intensive care unit on specialty support surfaces; this is likely an underestimation because it was not limited to those with SCI.[14] On air-fluidized beds, head-of-bed elevation greater than 15° increases shear on sacral and ischial flap sites.[5]

PRESSURE MAPPING

Pressure mapping is a technology that consists of a sensor mat that measures the pressure at the interface between the human body and a support surface, known as *interface pressure*.[15] Support surfaces include mattresses, commode seats, and wheelchair cushions. Pressure mapping systems also include a tablet that displays a color-coded image identifying surface contact and values of peak and average pressures (**Fig. 1**). Most systems, however, still require staff to manually find anatomic landmarks causing each area of pressure identified.[16]

CLINICAL USE

Pressure mapping is used in a variety of ways to evaluate different clinical goals of wound care management. First, it measures quantitative data (eg, peak pressures, average pressures, surface contact area, and time per position) to show relative differences in support surface performance to assist in the selection of the most clinically appropriate surface for each patient,[16,17] as differences in muscle bulk, skeletal frames, and body fat can influence interface pressure.[15,17] Pressure mapping used continuously informs providers and patients on pressure redistribution and decreases the prevalence of pressure injuries while in bed.[18–20] The real-time visual feedback is a

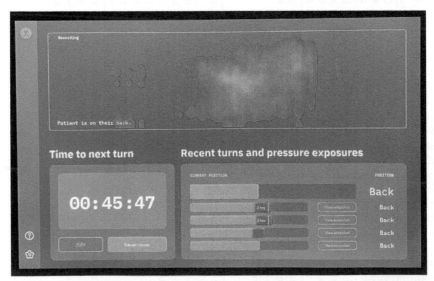

Fig. 1. *Pressure mapping display.* The Xsensor ForeSite Intelligent Surface displays an image of the body interface pressure, a turn timer, and history of turn positions. Actual pressure values are viewed by tapping the body image.

direct cue for patients to help direct their bed positioning and for providers to obtain maximum offloading.[18,20,21]

Importantly, the colors on a pressure map represent relative differences and are not absolute indicators of developing a pressure injury.[18] Although the values that colors represent are user-defined and influenced by research, "there is no proven relationship between the 32 mm Hg threshold and pressure ulcer susceptibility."[16,22] Many studies have reported benefits of using pressure mapping but caution its sole use due to other extrinsic and intrinsic factors that contribute to the development of pressure injuries, including temperature, moisture, friction, shear, and nutrition.[15,17] Furthermore, it is important to consider the reliability of the data based on the technology used and the environment where used. The quality of data can be influenced by the size of the pressure map, number of sensors in the mat, and sensitivity and resolution of the pressure values.[23] It is encouraged to use pressure mapping for identifying inappropriate support surfaces rather than creating a false sense of security on a support surface that maps well.[16]

CUSTOM CUSHIONS
Cushion Properties

Cushions for individuals who rely on wheeled mobility devices are an important aspect of wound care management. Wheelchair cushions are typically classified into 2 categories: positioning and skin protection.[24] For individuals with significant wound care concerns, the focus of a wheelchair cushion tends to lean toward skin protection, using fundamental properties of immersion and envelopment.[24] However, the most common skin protection cushions use air flotation, do not offer significant positional properties, and can be more fragile and complicated to properly use for patients who need positioning support.

Custom Cushion Technology

Custom cushion technology offers a comprehensive solution for individuals who need both significant positioning and skin protection. A custom negative cushion shape is created by molding the individual's pelvic anatomy and is converted to a unique, positive custom cushion. Custom cushions use orthotic principles of completely off-loading high-risk bony prominences of the pelvis (ischial tuberosities, sacrum/coccyx, and greater trochanters) to promote skin protection while loading areas with thicker tissue (proximal thighs and posterior lateral pelvis) to maintain positioning and stability. One study found that off-loading cushions reduced interface pressure under both the ischial tuberosities and the sacrum compared with air flotation style cushions in individuals with SCI.[25] The use of proper postural supports and off-loading shaped cushions has a positive effect on an individual's posture and treatment of stage 1 and 2 ischial tuberosity pressure injuries.[26] Many custom cushions are designed to minimize other extrinsic factors that contribute to skin breakdown: cushions and covers are breathable for temperature control, and custom shapes limit friction and shear. Although it is not the solution for all those at risk of pressure injuries, custom cushion technology can provide needed positioning support and off-loading properties to aid in wound care management.

IMAGING
Measuring Area

The manual approach for tracking wound size involves a ruler to measure the longest and widest dimensions. The elliptical model is a more elegant approach to calculate

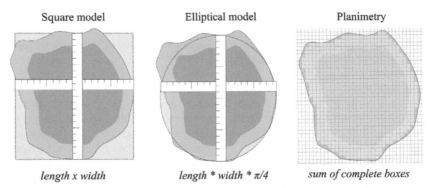

Fig. 2. *Approximating wound surface area.* The square and elliptical formulas estimate surface area (*denoted in blue*), useful for shallow wounds with simple shapes. Although time-consuming, planimetry yields the most accurate manual estimate. The utility of surface area is limited for large, complex wounds with varying depths, undermining, and tunneling.

the surface area via the formula length $\times$ width $\times$ $\pi/4$, yet it neither captures the complexity of large wounds (>40 cm^2) with varying depths and tissue infiltration nor removes interrater variability in measurement.[27]

Planimetry is a method in which the evaluator traces the wound over a transparent film, then using a superimposed grid counts the squares that fall within the tracing to estimate the wound surface area (**Fig. 2**). Although more accurate than linear measurements, it requires contact with the wound and is time-consuming. Digital planimetry is a hybrid approach in which software calculates the area of a manual tracing by integrating the pixels within the shape.[28]

Calculating Depth

Various algorithms have been developed to automate wound volume measurement from digital photographs more accurately than ruler-based methods. The first step is edge detection, which usually involves analyzing sudden changes in the intensity of pixels. From there, the area is calculated by integrating all pixels within the wound border.[29] The accuracy of this two-dimensional (2D) calculation is subject to variance from inconsistent body positioning and camera angles. Photo angle can be corrected using the data from an onboard gyroscope, a standard sensor on smart devices. However, limb curvature and positioning can still affect area calculations. Depth can be measured using "structure from motion" algorithms in which the depth of features is inferred from multiple images (or serial video frames) taken at varying angles. Stereophotogrammetry, in which the depth is derived from 2 cameras a fixed distance apart simultaneously taking photos,[30] is another approach to detecting depth from 2D content. Finally, laser technology can measure distance by calculating the time it takes for the laser to reflect off the wound surface and return to the sensor (**Fig. 3**).

Clinical Use

Although wound measurement (and more generally, feature detection) algorithms are well-described in computer vision literature,[29,30] commercialized devices have simplified the process with user-friendly software. Digital imaging is equally accurate and reliable as planimetry for determining area but systems using lasers to calculate volume have mixed results for accuracy and reliability.[28] A laser-assisted device

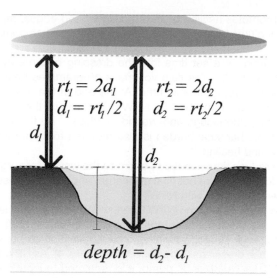

Fig. 3. *Depth measurement by laser.* This approach uses the speed of the laser light r, and the time t required to travel the round trip between emitter and tissue.

measured wound area accurately but consistently underestimated depth.[31] A longitudinal study found that three-dimensional measurements of diabetic foot ulcers had prognostic value for time to healing.[32]

Radiological Imaging

Wound examination at bedside is limited to visible tissue but imaging can portray the integrity of deeper structures. In our SCI practice, we are faced often with nonhealing chronic pressure injuries despite close follow-up, or sepsis due to pressure injury. Community-acquired pressure injuries overlying ischia are the most common in our patients with paralysis and tend to be deep with bony exposure. These scenarios are concerning for sinus tracts, abscesses, and osteomyelitis that can impede healing.

Various imaging modalities can identify deep infectious structures whose presence can drive clinical decision-making for wound care management. Plain films generally do not detect osteomyelitis during the first 2 weeks.[33] Three phase technetium bone scans have been shown to be highly sensitive (94%) and specific (95%) for osteomyelitis when radiographs were normal in pooled data from 6 studies but common findings near chronic wounds of bone remodeling and cellulitis compromise the ability to interpret these accurately. Leukocyte-labeled indium-111 scans can reveal osteomyelitis (85% sensitive and 88% specific in pooled data from 16 studies) and can be used with technetium scans.[34] Computed tomography can be used for diagnosing osteomyelitis, although MRI is the preferred modality (95% sensitive and 88% specific in pooled data from 11 studies).[34] We primarily use MRI in the workup to simultaneously plan debridement and myocutaneous flap closures.

Negative Pressure Wound Therapy

Negative pressure wound therapy (NPWT) and NPWT with instillation and dwell time (NPWTi-d) are 2 modalities for wounds of varied etiologies, including stage 3 and stage 4 pressure injuries often seen in those with SCIs. NPWT was approved for use in 1995 and promotes healing by contracting wound edges, removing bacteria, and reducing healing time by increasing granulation tissue when compared with other wound dressings.[35] In 2002, the additional ability to instill a fluid such as normal saline or a cleansing solution for a set time into the dressing became available to assist debridement of the wound.[35] The fluid volume is programmed based on the wound size, then dwells for a programmable time. At the end of the dwell time, the fluid is then suctioned from the wound bed by NPWT. This allows the fluid to dwell in the wound bed, liquefying the slough and wound exudate.[36] By flushing and cleansing the wound, planktonic bacterial burden is also reduced to create a more controlled environment for wound healing.[37]

This feature can reduce time needed to optimize the wound for surgical procedures, increase wound closures before hospital discharge, and generate less pain with dressing changes when compared with NPWT.[38]

There are some barriers to using NPWT and NPWTi-d. The skill level to place the dressings and operate the vacuum pumps can be complicated. Staff who care for patients with wounds require specific training in the application and operation of NPWT and NPWTi-d for these dressings to be successful[39] (**Fig. 4**). As NPWTi-d is only available with the V.A.C. ULTA (3M KCl) pump, it is restricted to inpatient use. High cost can also limit use.[37]

WOUND DRESSINGS
Skin Substitutes

Many different skin substitutes and matrices exist for chronic wound management for when other therapies have failed. The biologic types contain human cells (both neonatal and cadaver), or bovine and porcine cells. Nonbiologic or synthetic skin substitutes provide scaffolding for tissue growth and are similar to human extracellular matrix. Biologic skin substitutes contain a basement membrane and are more similar to native skin cells, which allows for more natural reepithelialization. Synthetic skin substitutes contain nonbiologic molecules and are biodegradable to provide scaffolding for reepithelialization.[40] Biologic skin substitutes have a higher risk of reaction than synthetic skin substitutes due to the increased risk of contamination. The major disadvantage of all skin substitutes is higher cost than traditional treatments and should be tried after other treatments have failed.[41]

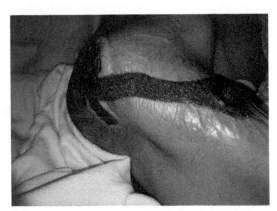

Fig. 4. NPWT applied to a pressure injury overlying the right greater trochanter. Note the bridging technique, in which the sponge dressing is extended anteriorly to avoid posterolateral pressure injury from the device's tubing.

Electrical Stimulation

Wounds naturally create changes in electrical potentials in the epidermis and dermis via diffusion of sodium from epidermis to dermis.[42] Fibroblasts, cells responsible for extracellular matrix deposition and remodeling,[43] have been shown to increase synthesis when electrically stimulated. Increased production of proteins like actin and integrin enhance fibroblast galvanotaxis,[42] or migration toward the electrical field, promoting extracellular matrix formation.

Typical electrical stimulation methods require the removal of the dressing and application of electrodes around the wound; thus stimulation occurs for a limited time and only within a clinical encounter. Multiple research groups have taken interest in designing wound dressings that integrate continuous electrical stimulation while a dressing covers a wound. Integrated designs generate current from the dressing itself, whereas exogenous designs use an external module to deliver current into the dressing. One integrated design (**Fig. 5**) contains a grid of alternating metallic (eg, silver and zinc) dots on the dressing that serves as cathodes and anodes of tiny batteries that generate microamperes via reduction–oxidation reactions in the presence of moisture.[44] The magnitude of current is similar to what is naturally produced.

Another dressing can remain in place for 7 days and deliver electrical stimulation continuously via an exogenous design (**Fig. 6**), which allows for the exchange of the power source module without disrupting the wound–dressing interface.[45,46] This dressing integrates sensors that record temperature and impedance to report the wound's health.

ULTRASOUND THERAPY

Noncontact, low-frequency ultrasound (NCLFU) is used in wound care to treat both chronic wounds and deep tissue pressure injuries (DTPIs). The ultrasonic device generates frequencies from 25 to 40 kHz to help remove devitalized tissue and

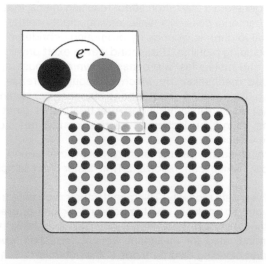

Fig. 5. Integrated design. Electrons (e⁻) flow from anodes to cathodes in the dressing to produce current.

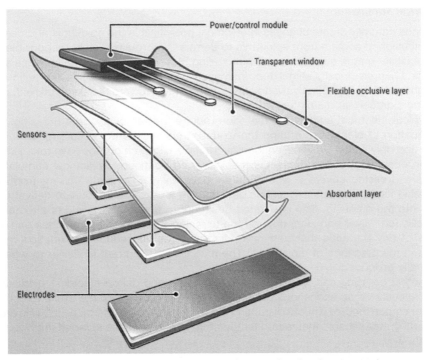

Fig. 6. Exogenous design. External module stimulates under the dressing and powers sensors. (Image created by Grace Gongaware.)

increase wound healing.[47] One commercial device (UltraMIST, SANUWAVE Health, Inc.) uses atomized normal saline vapor that acts as a transducer for the ultrasonic waves (**Fig. 7**) that generate a cavitation effect resulting in enzymatic fibrinolysis and the destruction of bacterial cell walls while leaving intact healthy structures.[47] This process is beneficial to chronic wounds by promoting debridement and decreasing bacterial burden including biofilms. Ultrasound waves exert physical forces on intracellular organelles and molecules, a process known as acoustic microstreaming[48] and is the proposed mechanism by which ultrasound increases growth factors, collagen production, vasodilation, macrophage responsiveness, and intracellular nitric oxide levels (that regulate inflammation). After treatments, a net efflux of intracellular calcium ions found in ischemic injuries contributes to restoration of homeostasis of the wound.[49]

NCLFU can also stimulate cellular activity below the wound injury surface to increase blood flow, which can resolve DTPIs faster than simply offloading the region.[49]

NCLFU is a relatively safe modality. The manufacturer recommends against the use of NCLFU near electronic implants and lumbosacral regions of pregnant women for theoretic risks, although to our knowledge, complications have not been demonstrated. It is contraindicated for malignant wounds, radiation wounds, those with thrombophlebitis, and bleeding disorders due to the potential increase in vasodilation and stimulation of cell growth.[47] A disadvantage of NCLFU is that its availability is usually limited to the hospital or clinic setting due to high cost.

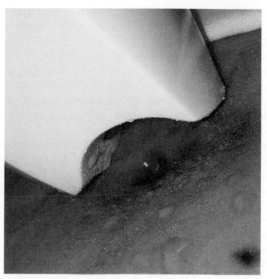

Fig. 7. *Ultrasound therapy application.* Saline mist transmits ultrasound waves to the tissue.

SUMMARY

Research in wound care management has led to advances in a wide array of technologies for prevention, monitoring, and treatment. The modalities discussed require clinical oversight and should be incorporated within the overall management plan by an interdisciplinary wound care team.

CLINICS CARE POINTS

- Patients at high risk for pressure injury should be placed on specialty mattresses and cushions to redistribute pressure between patient and surface, reduce shear, and control moisture.
- Wounds can be monitored using two-dimensional and three-dimensional models to approximate area and volume, respectively, whereas radiological studies can evaluate the involvement of structures deep to the visible wound bed.
- Negative pressure, electrical stimulation, and ultrasound therapies are means of promoting wound healing while skin substitutes provide scaffolding to facilitate re-epithelization.

DISCLOSURE

None of the authors has any financial disclosures to report, and they do not have any funding sources to report.

REFERENCES

1. Shah JB. The history of wound care. J Am Coll Certif Wound Spec 2011; 3(3):65–6.
2. McInnes E, Jammali-Blasi A, Bell-Syer SE, et al. Support surfaces for pressure ulcer prevention. Cochrane Wounds Group. Cochrane Database Syst Rev 2015. https://doi.org/10.1002/14651858.CD001735.pub5.

3. Kruger EA, Pires M, Ngann Y, et al. Comprehensive management of pressure ulcers in spinal cord injury: Current concepts and future trends. J Spinal Cord Med 2013;36(6):572–85.

4. McInnes E, Jammali-Blasi A, Bell-Syer SE, et al. Support surfaces for treating pressure ulcers. Cochrane Wounds Group. Cochrane Database Syst Rev 2018; 2018(10). https://doi.org/10.1002/14651858.CD009490.pub2.

5. Pressure Ulcer Prevention and Treatment Following Spinal Cord Injury: A Clinical Practice Guideline for Health-Care Professionals. J Spinal Cord Med 2001; 24(sup1):S40–101.

6. Moysidis T, Niebel W, Bartsch K, et al. Prevention of pressure ulcer: interaction of body characteristics and different mattresses. Int Wound J 2011;8(6):578–84.

7. European Pressure Ulcer Advisory Panel, National Pressure Injury Advisory Panel, Pan Pacific Pressure Injury Alliance. Prevention and treatment of pressure ulcers/injuries: Clinical practice guideline, The International Guideline. Haesler E, ed. EPUAP/NPIAP/PPPIA. Published online 2019.

8. Nixon J, Smith IL, Brown S, et al. Pressure Relieving Support Surfaces for Pressure Ulcer Prevention (PRESSURE 2): Clinical and Health Economic Results of a Randomised Controlled Trial. EClinicalMedicine 2019;14:42–52.

9. Finnegan MJ, Gazzerro L, Finnegan JO, et al. Comparing the effectiveness of a specialized alternating air pressure mattress replacement system and an air-fluidized integrated bed in the management of post-operative flap patients: A randomized controlled pilot study. J Tissue Viability 2008;17(1):2–9.

10. Mendoza RA, Lorusso GA, Ferrer DA, et al. A prospective, randomised controlled trial evaluating the effectiveness of the fluid immersion simulation system vs an air-fluidised bed system in the acute postoperative management of pressure ulcers: A midpoint study analysis. Int Wound J 2019;16(4):989–99.

11. Marchione FG, Araújo LMQ, Araújo LV. Approaches that use software to support the prevention of pressure ulcer: A systematic review. Int J Med Inf 2015;84(10): 725–36.

12. Tran JP, McLaughlin JM, Li RT, et al. Prevention of Pressure Ulcers in the Acute Care Setting: New Innovations and Technologies. Plast Reconstr Surg 2016; 138:232S–40S.

13. Goetz LL, Brown GS, Priebe MM. Interface Pressure Characteristics Of Alternating Air Cell Mattresses In Persons With Spinal Cord Injury. J Spinal Cord Med 2002;25(3):167–73.

14. Ooka M, Kemp MG, McMyn R, et al. Evaluation of three types of support surfaces for preventing pressure ulcers in patients in a surgical intensive care unit. J Wound Ostomy Cont Nurs 1995;22(6):271–9.

15. Barnett RI, Shelton FE. Measurement of support surface efficacy: pressure. Adv Wound Care 1997;10(7):21–9.

16. Jan YK, Brienza D. Technology for Pressure Ulcer Prevention. Top Spinal Cord Inj Rehabil 2006;11(4):30–41.

17. Shelton F, Barnett R, Meyer E. Full-body interface pressure testing as a method for performance evaluation of clinical support surfaces. Appl Ergon 1998;29(6): 491–7.

18. Gunningberg L, Carli C. Reduced pressure for fewer pressure ulcers: can real-time feedback of interface pressure optimise repositioning in bed? Int Wound J 2016;13(5):774–9.

19. Behrendt R, Ghaznavi AM, Mahan M, et al. Continuous Bedside Pressure Mapping and Rates of Hospital-Associated Pressure Ulcers in a Medical Intensive Care Unit. Am J Crit Care 2014;23(2):127–33.

20. Gammon HM, Shelton CB, Siegert C, et al. Self-turning for pressure injury prevention. Wound Med 2016;12:15–8.
21. Scott RG, Thurman KM. Visual Feedback of Continuous Bedside Pressure Mapping to Optimize Effective Patient Repositioning. Adv Wound Care 2014;3(5): 376–82.
22. Brienza DM, Karg PE, Jo Geyer M, et al. The relationship between pressure ulcer incidence and buttock-seat cushion interface pressure in at-risk elderly wheelchair users. Arch Phys Med Rehabil 2001;82(4):529–33.
23. Eitzen I. Pressure mapping in seating: a frequency analysis approach. Arch Phys Med Rehabil 2004;85(7):1136–40.
24. Brienza D, Kelsey S, Karg P, et al. A randomized clinical trial on preventing pressure ulcers with wheelchair seat cushions. J Am Geriatr Soc 2010;58(12): 2308–14.
25. Crane B, Wininger M, Call E. Orthotic-Style Off-Loading Wheelchair Seat Cushion Reduces Interface Pressure Under Ischial Tuberosities and Sacrococcygeal Regions. Arch Phys Med Rehabil 2016;97(11):1872–9.
26. Crivelli N, Cafueri G, Zucchiatti N. Italian Journal of Prevention, Diagnostic and Therapeutic Medicine. ijpdtm 2021;4(1):72–80.
27. Bowling FL, KIng L, Fadavi H, et al. An assessment of the accuracy and usability of a novel optical wound measurement system. Diabet Med J Br Diabet Assoc 2009;26(1):93–6.
28. Jørgensen LB, Sørensen JA, Jemec GB, et al. Methods to assess area and volume of wounds - a systematic review: Review of methods to assess wound size. Int Wound J 2016;13(4):540–53.
29. Galperin YV. An image processing Tour of College Mathematics. 1st edition. New York, NY: Chapman & Hall, CRC Press; 2020.
30. Liu C, Fan X, Guo Z, et al. Wound area measurement with 3D transformation and smartphone images. BMC Bioinformatics 2019;20(1):724.
31. Davis KE, Constantine FC, Macaslan EC, et al. Validation of a laser-assisted wound measurement device for measuring wound volume. J Diabetes Sci Technol 2013;7(5):1161–6.
32. Malone M, Schwarzer S, Walsh A, et al. Monitoring wound progression to healing in diabetic foot ulcers using three-dimensional wound imaging. J Diabetes Complications 2020;34(2):107471.
33. Ruan CM, Escobedo E, Harrison S, et al. Magnetic resonance imaging of non-healing pressure ulcers and myocutaneous flaps. Arch Phys Med Rehabil 1998;79(9):1080–8.
34. Schauwecker DS. The scintigraphic diagnosis of osteomyelitis. AJR Am J Roentgenol 1992;158(1):9–18.
35. Faust E, Opoku-Agyeman JL, Behnam AB. Use of Negative-Pressure Wound Therapy With Instillation and Dwell Time: An Overview. Plast Reconstr Surg 2021;147(1S-1):16S–26S.
36. Crumley C. Negative Pressure Wound Therapy Devices With Instillation/Irrigation: A Technologic Analysis. J Wound Ostomy Continence Nurs 2021;48(3):199–202.
37. Fletcher J, Mosahebi A, Younis I, et al. Negative pressure wound therapy with instillation for Category 3 and 4 pressure ulcers: Findings of an advisory board meeting. Wounds UK 2019;15(3):72–7.
38. Gupta S, Gabriel A, Lantis J, et al. Clinical recommendations and practical guide for negative pressure wound therapy with instillation. Int Wound J 2016;13(2): 159–74.

39. Cray A. Negative pressure wound therapy and nurse education. Br J Nurs 2017; 26(15):S6–18.
40. Halim A, Khoo T, Shah JY. Biologic and synthetic skin substitutes: An overview. Indian J Plast Surg 2010;43(3):23.
41. Varnado M. Skin substitutes: understanding product differences: choosing the right product can prove critical to patient care–and to staff resources in a busy clinic. Wound Care Advis 2016;5(6):30+.
42. Ennis WJ, Lee C, Gellada K, et al. Advanced Technologies to Improve Wound Healing: Electrical Stimulation, Vibration Therapy, and Ultrasound-What Is the Evidence? Plast Reconstr Surg 2016;138(3 Suppl):94S–104S.
43. desJardins-Park HE, Foster DS, Longaker MT. Fibroblasts and wound healing: an update. Regen Med 2018;13(5):491–5.
44. Yu C, Hu ZQ, Peng RY. Effects and mechanisms of a microcurrent dressing on skin wound healing: a review. Mil Med Res 2014;1:24.
45. Scalamandré A, Bogie KM. Smart technologies in wound prevention and care. In: Amit Gefen, editor. Innovations and Emerging technologies in wound care. Academic Press; 2020. p. 225–44. https://doi.org/10.1016/B978-0-12-815028-3.00013-4.
46. Bogie KM, Garverick S, Zorman CA, et al. Integrated surface stimulation device for wound therapy and infection control. Available at: https://patents.google.com/patent/US10201703B2. Accessed October 1, 2021.
47. Ramundo J, Gray M. Is Ultrasonic Mist Therapy Effective for Debriding Chronic Wounds? J Wound Ostomy Continence Nurs 2008;35(6):579–83.
48. Johns LD. Nonthermal effects of therapeutic ultrasound: the frequency resonance hypothesis. J Athl Train 2002;37(3):293–9.
49. Wagner-Cox P, Duhame HM, Jamison CR, et al. Use of Noncontact Low-Frequency Ultrasound in Deep Tissue Pressure Injury: A Retrospective Analysis. J Wound Ostomy Continence Nurs 2017;44(4):336–42.

UNITED STATES POSTAL SERVICE ®

Statement of Ownership, Management, and Circulation
(All Periodicals Publications Except Requester Publications)

1. Publication Title	2. Publication Number	3. Filing Date
PHYSICAL MEDICINE AND REHABILITATION CLINICS	009 – 243	9/18/2022

4. Issue Frequency	5. Number of Issues Published Annually	6. Annual Subscription Price
FEB, MAY, AUG, NOV	4	$332.00

7. Complete Mailing Address of Known Office of Publication (Not printer) (Street, city, county, state, and ZIP+4®)

ELSEVIER INC.
230 Park Avenue, Suite 800
New York, NY 10169

Contact Person
Malathi Samayan

Telephone (Include area code)
91-44-4289-4507

8. Complete Mailing Address of Headquarters or General Business Office of Publisher (Not printer)

ELSEVIER INC.
230 Park Avenue, Suite 800
New York, NY 10169

9. Full Names and Complete Mailing Addresses of Publisher, Editor, and Managing Editor (Do not leave blank)

Publisher (Name and complete mailing address)

Dolores Meloni, ELSEVIER INC.
1600 JOHN F KENNEDY BLVD. SUITE 1800
PHILADELPHIA, PA 19103-2899

Editor (Name and complete mailing address)

Megan Ashdown, ELSEVIER INC.
1600 JOHN F KENNEDY BLVD. SUITE 1800
PHILADELPHIA, PA 19103-2899

Managing Editor (Name and complete mailing address)

PATRICK MANLEY, ELSEVIER INC.
1600 JOHN F KENNEDY BLVD. SUITE 1800
PHILADELPHIA, PA 19103-2899

10. Owner (Do not leave blank. If the publication is owned by a corporation, give the name and address of the corporation immediately followed by the names and addresses of all stockholders owning or holding 1 percent or more of the total amount of stock. If not owned by a corporation, give the names and addresses of the individual owners. If owned by a partnership or other unincorporated firm, give its name and address as well as those of each individual owner. If the publication is published by a nonprofit organization, give its name and address.)

Full Name	Complete Mailing Address
WHOLLY OWNED SUBSIDIARY OF REED/ELSEVIER, US HOLDINGS	1600 JOHN F KENNEDY BLVD. SUITE 1800 PHILADELPHIA, PA 19103-2899

11. Known Bondholders, Mortgagees, and Other Security Holders Owning or Holding 1 Percent or More of Total Amount of Bonds, Mortgages, or Other Securities. If none, check box ▶ ☐ None

Full Name	Complete Mailing Address
N/A	

12. Tax Status (For completion by nonprofit organizations authorized to mail at nonprofit rates) (Check one)
The purpose, function, and nonprofit status of this organization and the exempt status for federal income tax purposes:
☒ Has Not Changed During Preceding 12 Months
☐ Has Changed During Preceding 12 Months (Publisher must submit explanation of change with this statement)

PS Form **3526**, July 2014 [Page 1 of 4 (see instructions page 4)] PSN: 7530-01-000-9931   PRIVACY NOTICE: See our privacy policy on www.usps.com.

---

13. Publication Title	14. Issue Date for Circulation Data Below
PHYSICAL MEDICINE AND REHABILITATION CLINICS OF NORTH AMERICA	MAY 2022

15. Extent and Nature of Circulation		Average No. Copies Each Issue During Preceding 12 Months	No. Copies of Single Issue Published Nearest to Filing Date
a. Total Number of Copies (Net press run)		179	161
b. Paid Circulation (By Mail and Outside the Mail)	(1) Mailed Outside-County Paid Subscriptions Stated on PS Form 3541 (Include paid distribution above nominal rate, advertiser's proof copies, and exchange copies)	93	84
	(2) Mailed In-County Paid Subscriptions Stated on PS Form 3541 (Include paid distribution above nominal rate, advertiser's proof copies, and exchange copies)	0	0
	(3) Paid Distribution Outside the Mails Including Sales Through Dealers and Carriers, Street Vendors, Counter Sales, and Other Paid Distribution Outside USPS®	41	24
	(4) Paid Distribution by Other Classes of Mail Through the USPS (e.g., First-Class Mail®)	0	0
c. Total Paid Distribution (Sum of 15b (1), (2), (3), and (4))	▶	134	108
d. Free or Nominal Rate Distribution (By Mail and Outside the Mail)	(1) Free or Nominal Rate Outside-County Copies included on PS Form 3541	26	34
	(2) Free or Nominal Rate In-County Copies included on PS Form 3541	0	0
	(3) Free or Nominal Rate Copies Mailed at Other Classes Through the USPS (e.g., First-Class Mail)	0	0
	(4) Free or Nominal Rate Distribution Outside the Mail (Carriers or other means)	0	0
e. Total Free or Nominal Rate Distribution (Sum of 15d (1), (2), (3) and (4))	▶	26	34
f. Total Distribution (Sum of 15c and 15e)	▶	160	142
g. Copies not Distributed (See Instructions to Publishers #4 (page #3))	▶	19	19
h. Total (Sum of 15f and g)	▶	179	161
i. Percent Paid (15c divided by 15f times 100)		83.75%	76.05%

* If you are claiming electronic copies, go to line 16 on page 3. If you are not claiming electronic copies, skip to line 17 on page 3.

PS Form **3526**, July 2014 (Page 2 of 4)

16. Electronic Copy Circulation		Average No. Copies Each Issue During Preceding 12 Months	No. Copies of Single Issue Published Nearest to Filing Date
a. Paid Electronic Copies	▶		
b. Total Paid Print Copies (Line 15c) + Paid Electronic Copies (Line 16a)	▶		
c. Total Print Distribution (Line 15f) + Paid Electronic Copies (Line 16a)	▶		
d. Percent Paid (Both Print & Electronic Copies) (16b divided by 16c × 100)	▶		

☒ I certify that 50% of all my distributed copies (electronic and print) are paid above a nominal price.

17. Publication of Statement of Ownership

☒ If the publication is a general publication, publication of this statement is required. Will be printed in the **NOVEMBER 2022** issue of this publication.   ☐ Publication not required.

18. Signature and Title of Editor, Publisher, Business Manager, or Owner

Malathi Samayan   Date 9/18/2022

Malathi Samayan - Distribution Controller

I certify that all information furnished on this form is true and complete. I understand that anyone who furnishes false or misleading information on this form or who omits material or information requested on the form may be subject to criminal sanctions (including fines and imprisonment) and/or civil sanctions (including civil penalties).

PS Form **3526**, July 2014 (Page 3 of 4)   PRIVACY NOTICE: See our privacy policy on www.usps.com.

Moving?

Make sure your subscription moves with you!

To notify us of your new address, find your **Clinics Account Number** (located on your mailing label above your name), and contact customer service at:

Email: journalscustomerservice-usa@elsevier.com

800-654-2452 (subscribers in the U.S. & Canada)
314-447-8871 (subscribers outside of the U.S. & Canada)

Fax number: 314-447-8029

Elsevier Health Sciences Division
Subscription Customer Service
3251 Riverport Lane
Maryland Heights, MO 63043

*To ensure uninterrupted delivery of your subscription, please notify us at least 4 weeks in advance of move.